THE BUDGET-FRIENDLY Fresh and Local
DIABETES COOKBOOK

By Charles Mattocks, "The Poor Chef"

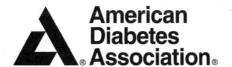

American Diabetes Association.

Director, Book Publishing, Abe Ogden; *Managing Editor,* Greg Guthrie; *Acquisitions Editor,* Victor Van Beuren; *Editor,* Lauren Wilson; *Production Manager,* Melissa Sprott; *Composition,* Circle Graphics; *Cover Design,* Jenn French Designs, LLC; *Photographer,* Renee Comet Photography; *Printer,* RR Donnelley.

Printed in the United States of America
1 3 5 7 9 10 8 6 4 2

The suggestions and information contained in this publication are generally consistent with the *Clinical Practice Recommendations* and other policies of the American Diabetes Association, but they do not represent the policy or position of the Association or any of its boards or committees. Reasonable steps have been taken to ensure the accuracy of the information presented. However, the American Diabetes Association cannot ensure the safety or efficacy of any product or service described in this publication. Individuals are advised to consult a physician or other appropriate health care professional before undertaking any diet or exercise program or taking any medication referred to in this publication. Professionals must use and apply their own professional judgment, experience, and training and should not rely solely on the information contained in this publication before prescribing any diet, exercise, or medication. The American Diabetes Association—its officers, directors, employees, volunteers, and members—assumes no responsibility or liability for personal or other injury, loss, or damage that may result from the suggestions or information in this publication.

♾ The paper in this publication meets the requirements of the ANSI Standard Z39.48-1992 (permanence of paper).

ADA titles may be purchased for business or promotional use or for special sales. To purchase more than 50 copies of this book at a discount, or for custom editions of this book with your logo, contact the American Diabetes Association at the address below, at booksales@diabetes.org, or by calling 703-299-2046.

American Diabetes Association
1701 North Beauregard Street
Alexandria, Virginia 22311

DOI: 10.2337/9781580405119

Library of Congress Cataloging-in-Publication Data
Mattocks, Charles.
  The budget-friendly fresh and local diabetes cookbook / Charles Mattocks, The Poor Chef.
     pages cm
  Includes bibliographical references and index.
  ISBN 978-1-58040-511-9 (alk. paper)
  1. Diabetes--Diet therapy--Recipes. 2. Diabetes--Economic aspects. I. Title.
  RC662.M358 2014
  641.5'6314--dc23
                         2013036475

This book is dedicated to my mom, Constance Marley,
and my little girls, Elle and Izzy.
The true joys of my life.

Table of Contents

Acknowledgments

First and foremost, I would like to thank my team. When I started this dream of saving lives, I knew I needed dedicated, hard-working people to join me. They are the ones who help me keep fighting.

Many thanks to:

The great people along this journey who have allowed me to keep the faith. Julia Begg and John Molson, Ken and the Syntra 5 team, Dave at Great West Van's. Martina Desgouttes of Healthy Explosion for her wealth of knowledge, passion for health, abiding faith, and for always knowing just what to say to uplift us. Katherine Tomlinson for her invaluable input. Junior Farrell for being an amazing friend and brother. The Jamaican Diabetes Association. Shawn and his family. The International Diabetes Federation for their support. Kelly Hall, Deb Scott, John Wallace, and Tai and her new baby. My little sister Shayna and my dad, who I truly love, Dadalni Mattocks.

My son and best friend, Armani, who was the main reason I started down this path to begin with. Junior from Jamaica. Constance Marley, my lovely mother, who is the strongest woman I know. My designer, Terry "the amazing man" Hicks, for having my back and for making sure my artwork and designs are always amazing. Justin Gardner from Shire for helping us journey to India and for trusting in the dream even in its earliest stages. Bernis from Heal Together for helping my RV get on the road.

Victor Van Beuren from the American Diabetes Association for giving me the chance to share my recipes and thoughts. Thanks to Alicia Boucher. Vicki Schmelzer. My brother Drew

Marley. John Ost. Tiana Marie and her lil daughter. My cousins Prince and Alex "the rebel" Marley. Michel Cooper and the Cooper family. David Samuel, Joel Francois, and Shawn Epperson. My neighbor and friend Juan and his family. Joyce (aka LJ). Lisa Summers and Roger. My brother Andrew Livingston. Rick Williams. Dr. Steven Bloom, Dr. Desmond Bell, Jeff Frenchman, Marc Brissett, and Chef Theo Plowden. Zack "attacks" and his mom and their struggle with type 1— keep changing lives! Jeff at Total Wellness. Personalabs. Chef to the stars Dolores Murgatroyd. Brian Buckley. Dr. Bowman. Traenne. Brother Douglas Gooden for being a strong force in this mission and a great brother. Maria and her son Zay for always being there and fighting this battle with me. A big thanks to "TV" Terence Noonan for giving me some great opportunities, and the staff at Dr. Oz and Anderson Cooper. To my friends from Elmont Long Island, Facebook, and Twitter. Kathleen Lane. Duran and his lovely wife, Arif, and mother. Kurtis. Monika Mcglon and Maya, Benni, and Jasmina Mattocks for holding me down for many years. Rohan, and Cedella Marley. Julie Dubois. Curwin Callender. My new family in Trinidad: Auntie Pam and her lovely daughters, Nikki, T, Kim, and Kathy. Auntie Alma and Amanda, her daughter from Canada. Otto from cnc3. Rosanna from Trini. I am sure there are more and I could go on for days but these are the core of who I am now. Much love to all! I hope you've enjoyed this journey with me.

And, of course, to everyone living with diabetes. You also are a part of this team. I hope these recipes will be a start to a healthier you. You deserve the quality, freshness, and nutrition found in the products from your farmers markets. As the past generations have helped us may we help the ones who follow us. May what we learn about healthy minds, bodies, and spirits enrich our children and our children's children. I look forward to a brighter future for all of us. I am honored to travel this road with you.

Foreword

"I won't ever be able to eat anything that tastes good again! I will have to worry about all the possible complications of this disease and I won't even be able to have the enjoyment of a good meal!" This was the cry of a woman who talked to me at an American Diabetes Association event several days after she had been diagnosed with diabetes. I understood her concern. I felt the same way after my diagnosis. I loved to cook and I loved to eat. I thought having diabetes meant that I would have a lifetime of bland, tasteless meals.

I was able to assure this woman that dishes like mouth-watering Thai Chicken Kabobs, Crunchy Chopped Salad, and Tropical Fruit Mousse could all be part of affordable, healthy, diabetes-friendly cuisine. And the biggest payoff is that eating these meals may help us avoid the complications of diabetes.

For years I have enjoyed occasional trips to farmers markets. After my diagnosis I realized how many diabetes-friendly ingredients could be found there. The recipes you will find in this book will be full of those ingredients. Fresh, local, healthy, and delicious—those are the kinds of foods I have included in my book…our book!

This book is for all of my fellow citizens in the world of diabetes. There are some important rules in our new world. Our lives depend on learning and following those rules. But it's worth it because we are worth it.

My diagnosis came as a complete shock to me. I thought I was in great health. I actually did not know a lot about diabetes before my diagnosis. The more I have learned, the more I have realized the importance of being an advocate for diabetes education, prevention, and research in order to stem the tide of this disease.

Here are some diabetes "rules of the road" to keep in mind:

+ Eat a breakfast that combines complex carbs with protein (e.g., whole-wheat toast with peanut butter, oatmeal with nuts and fruit, poached eggs and a whole-wheat English muffin).
+ Eat a variety of colorful fruits and vegetables. A rule of thumb: the more vibrant the color, the higher the nutritional value.
+ Use herbs and spices to enhance the flavors of your foods.
+ Give your taste buds time to adjust to new tastes and textures. It may take a little while for you to get used to natural flavors when they are no longer masked by added sugar and salt.

Feel free to be adventurous within these guidelines. Prepare a breakfast dish for dinner. Have a salad as a dinner. Enjoy an icy, vitamin C–filled fruit drink as a dessert. I offer you these recipes to use as you desire. Think of them as tools to use as you work to maintain your health and realize your dreams.

And now that we have a few of the rules, let's start our journey through a book that will make your life with diabetes easier and tastier.

Me, My Diabetes, and My Uncle Bob

My uncle taught me that it was not my right to dream big, it was my obligation. Years ago, as I listened to him in my mother's apartment in New York, I accepted this challenge as my birthright.

Others might have looked at this man and noticed how his hair was falling out or how his thin skin seemed to be stretched taut over his high cheekbones. But I noticed the fire in his eyes and I focused on the words he spoke over me like a blessing: "There is only one person who can make you a failure…the person who stares back at you from the mirror." This man, determined to fight disease, recognized in me something that no one else did. He saw my passion to make a difference. It was his passion and determination that drove my uncle to create songs such as "Buffalo Soldier" and "Redemption Song." That day I learned lessons that would change my life. They were taught to me by my uncle Bob Marley.

Self-fulfilling prophecies of failure can try to worm their way into our thoughts and destroy who we were meant to be. Who can change that? In the words of my uncle, "Emancipate yourselves from mental slavery; none but ourselves can free our minds." I took those words to heart and set out to work toward my dreams. I had a measure of success and felt good about it. Then I was diagnosed with type 2 diabetes. I felt that my body had turned against me. What good was success when I had a disease I would have to deal with every day for the rest of my life? Angrily, I tried to push that lesson from my uncle away, but it kept coming back. Now I am following his imperative to "conquer the devils with a little thing called love." We are fighting the "devil" of diabetes and we are doing it with hard work and lots of love. That fight, my friends, begins in our own minds and our own homes.

I wish there was a cure for diabetes. I wish we didn't have to check our numbers, be so careful about what we eat, or take insulin or other meds. I wish diabetes didn't cause people to lose their sight, their limbs, or their lives. But I know that until a cure is found we must check those numbers, watch what we eat, and follow the advice of our doctors. That will help us keep our vision, keep our feet and legs, and live longer lives.

My uncle Bob once said, "Open your eyes, look within. Are you satisfied with the life you are living?" I will be honest with you, some days I am not satisfied with how I am living. I wish I could be a "better" diabetes patient. Sometimes I binge on things I know I should not eat. I admit sometimes I don't exercise as often as I should. Sometimes I don't check my numbers regularly or get enough rest or follow the advice I give to other people with diabetes.

Sometimes I just want to pull the covers up over my head and pretend that I don't have diabetes. I have my pity party, I indulge myself in a little bit of negative thinking, and then I get up and start all over again. Bottom line: I want to live. And I want you to live too. I cannot tell you to do what I am not willing to do. So join me and move from saying "I wish" to "I do."

I do know I have to be kind to myself. I have to forgive myself when I fall, get up quickly, and make better choices. So do you. *I do* know that checking my numbers is essential to knowing just how my body is processing what I eat. So do you.

I do know that eating healthier will make me feel better mentally and physically. So do you.

I do know that I will continue on this journey as long as I am able. I hope to see you along the way.

Welcome To My Kitchen

The kitchen has always been my favorite room of the house. It's a place for families to work together, laugh together, and enjoy each other's company as they create the foods that will nourish and sustain them. The scents of allspice and roasting chicken take me back in time to the warmth and comfort of my grandmother's kitchen. I watched as she measured a "pinch" of this and a "handful" of that. If I behaved well, I was allowed the first taste of whatever creation she was preparing. "Is it good?" she would ask. Of course it was always good!

In my mother's kitchen I learned to be more precise as I helped measure with cups and teaspoons. Often I would be home from school before my mother returned from work. I took pride in being able to have the supper ready before she walked in the door. "Is it good?" I would ask her. And, just about always, she said it was good. When it wasn't, she took the time to teach me how to do better.

When I became a single dad, I would pull a chair up to the counter for my son to stand on. He helped me measure—some pinches, some teaspoons and cups. When we sat down to eat he would grin and say, "I helped and it tastes so good."

My son is the person who encouraged me to become the "Poor Chef." My diagnosis of type 2 diabetes has inspired me to add "Diabetes Advocate" to that title. The realities of diabetes may have changed my food choices, and yours, but we can improve our recipes and our health by using fresh local ingredients.

Your kitchen can still be the center of your home. Involve your children in planning, shopping for, and preparing meals. Taking your children to the farmers market with you can become something to look forward to each week. Let them choose a new fruit or vegetable to try or help you pick out a new recipe that will include what you have purchased. They will be much more willing to try something new if they are part of the process of bringing it to the table.

There are many differences between my grandmother's kitchen, my mother's kitchen, and mine but there is one constant. That constant is love. And no matter how we may have to adjust our diets, that love is what makes your kitchen and mine very special.

Positive Affirmations

We always hear, "You are what you eat." I agree with that completely. But, let's take that a step further: "You are what you believe." This is another essential part of a healthy life. Let's call it Vitamin P for Vitamin Positivity! Don't tell yourself that you will be healthier in the future. Claim it now!

Look in the mirror each morning and say, "This is a great day! I am someone who is worthy of all good things and good health is mine."

Then go out there and live your life as if it is true and so it will be.

Today I *refuse* to let unhealthy foods or thoughts enter my body, mind, or spirit. Today I *choose* to honor my body, mind, and spirit with only that which is for my highest good.

W ake up! I don't need an alarm clock to give that message to me in the morning. I wake up, usually very early, ready to get back to work on the mission that has become my life: building up people with diabetes so together we can tear down this disease. This mission takes commitment and it takes energy. That energy, in the form of a healthy breakfast, is needed first thing in the morning to "break the fast" and get your body going. You could say that your first meal of the day is your metabolism's alarm clock.

So what should we eat at the beginning of the day? Often I will have a smoothie full of fruit, low-fat yogurt, and some protein powder. When I have more time I like to prepare one of the dishes I have included in this breakfast section.

I can hear you now: "What about the carbs? I see carbs in there." Let me say this: not long after I was diagnosed with type 2 diabetes I met a man who had lived with the disease for ten years. "Charles," he said, "carb is not one of those four letter words you aren't supposed to say. Moderation. Just remember moderation."

I met with a nutritionist after I was diagnosed. I asked dozens of questions and received dozens of answers. She recommended books and websites and I continue to search for new answers every day. In her advice to me, she echoed that word "moderation." We need to carefully plan our meals. It shouldn't be a burden. We should see it as a way of honoring ourselves and our bodies.

One of the many reasons I love shopping at farmers markets is because I know the ingredients there will help me honor my body. They are fresh. They haven't traveled miles and miles to get to me. The stand holders are proud to offer them for sale. And I am proud to support farmers markets wherever I travel.

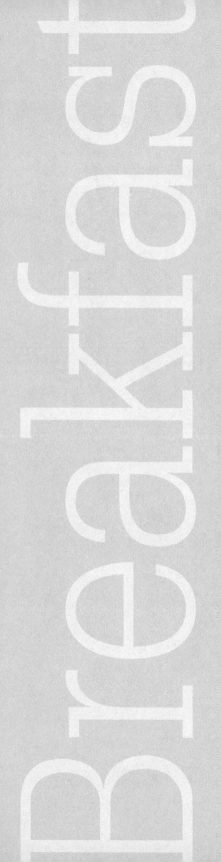

Scrambled Eggs with Salmon and Dill

Crustless Quiche with Veggies

Salmon Hash

"Loaded" Oatmeal with Ginger, Sunflower Seeds, and Chopped Dried Apricots

Banana Split Breakfast Smoothie

Nuts about Pizza for Breakfast

Chicken and the Egg Omelette

Sweet and Smoky Baked Eggs

Applesauce Pancakes

Savory Breakfast Egg Custard

Breakfast Baked Apples

Peach Melba Smoothie

Delish Deviled Eggs

Scrambled Eggs with Salmon and Dill

SERVES 4

SERVING SIZE 1/4th recipe

1 Tbsp	olive oil
4 oz	leftover salmon
1	egg
1	egg white
2 Tbsp	milk (non-fat is fine)
1 tsp	ground white pepper
2 Tbsp	fresh dill (or 1 tsp dried dill)

1 Heat the olive oil in a medium skillet. Shred the salmon into small pieces.

2 Whisk together the egg, egg white, milk, and seasonings. Add the fish to the eggs.

3 Pour egg mixture into hot skillet. Using a spatula, push the egg around so that the cooked parts are constantly being moved to the center of the skillet.

4 Remove from heat when the eggs are glossy. They'll continue cooking on the plate, so don't let them get too dry.

CHEF'S NOTES: My original, before-diabetes recipe called for smoked salmon or lox. Using leftover cooked salmon or canned salmon will cut down the amount of sodium in this dish but not one bit of the flavor.

Exchanges/Food Choices
1 Lean Meat   1 Fat

Basic Nutritional Values

Calories	105	
Calories from Fat	65	
Total Fat	7.0	g
Saturated Fat	1.3	g
Trans Fat	0.0	g
Cholesterol	65	mg
Sodium	50	mg
Potassium	130	mg
Total Carbohydrate	1	g
Dietary Fiber	0	g
Sugars	1	g
Protein	9	g
Phosphorus	100	mg

Crustless Quiche with Veggies

SERVES 6

1 Tbsp	olive oil
1	medium purple onion, finely chopped
1	medium zucchini, finely chopped
1 cup	broccoli florets, finely chopped
1	large egg, lightly beaten
4	egg whites, lightly beaten
½ cup	low-fat (1%) milk
3 Tbsp	flour
1 Tbsp	grated reduced-fat Parmesan cheese
¼ cup	grated reduced-fat sharp cheddar cheese
1 tsp	garlic powder
Dash	salt and pepper
Dash	hot sauce (optional)

1 Preheat oven to 350°F.

2 In nonstick frying pan heat oil, add veggies, and cook until crisp/tender.

3 In a large bowl mix eggs, egg whites, milk, flour, cheeses, and seasonings. Add cooked veggies and stir.

4 Pour into lightly greased pie plate or shallow casserole dish. Bake 30–35 minutes or until set.

CHEF'S NOTES: Be creative when it comes to the veggies you add to this. When I have leftover cooked vegetables in my fridge I like to experiment with different combinations. As far as the hot sauce, well, you know that is not optional for me!

Exchanges/Food Choices
1 Vegetable   1 Medium-Fat Meat

Basic Nutritional Values

Calories	90
Calories from Fat	40
Total Fat	4.5 g
Saturated Fat	1.4 g
Trans Fat	0.0 g
Cholesterol	35 mg
Sodium	125 mg
Potassium	250 mg
Total Carbohydrate	6 g
Dietary Fiber	1 g
Sugars	3 g
Protein	7 g
Phosphorus	105 mg

Salmon Hash

½ lb   red potatoes, unpeeled
2 Tbsp   olive oil
1   small purple onion, chopped
½ cup   fresh salsa
½ tsp   salt
2 Tbsp   fresh dill
¾ lb   cooked salmon, broken into small
pieces

1. Steam potatoes and cut into cubes.

2. Heat olive oil in large, nonstick frying pan. Add onions and cook until they soften.

3. Add salsa and other ingredients and cook over medium-high heat until mixture is crisp on the bottom. Flip with spatula and brown the other side.

4. Serve with a poached egg on top (optional).

CHEF'S NOTES: I like to prepare my own salsa with lots of cilantro. Use your favorite version. If you use jarred salsa be sure to check the label to make certain you are not adding sugar and empty calories to this dish.

Exchanges/Food Choices
1 Starch   3 Lean Meat   1 1/2 Fat

Basic Nutritional Values

Calories	275
Calories from Fat	125
Total Fat	14.0 g
Saturated Fat	2.3 g
Trans Fat	0.0 g
Cholesterol	60 mg
Sodium	525 mg
Potassium	605 mg
Total Carbohydrate	15 g
Dietary Fiber	2 g
Sugars	3 g
Protein	21 g
Phosphorus	235 mg

"Loaded" Oatmeal with Ginger, Sunflower Seeds, and Chopped Dried Apricots

SERVES 4

1 cup	rolled oats
3/4 cup	unsweetened coconut milk beverage/drink
1 1/4 cup	nonfat milk
1 tsp	ground ginger
1/3 cup	chopped dried apricots
2 Tbsp	unsalted sunflower seeds

1 Combine all ingredients in a heavy saucepan. Bring to a boil, stirring occasionally.

2 Turn down to a simmer.

3 Cook about 10 minutes until thickened.

CHEF'S NOTES: I love to experiment with different add-ins for my oatmeal. Try adding dried fruit while cooking or fresh fruit after the oatmeal is done. Toss in some seeds or nuts to add even more fiber and nutrients.

Exchanges/Food Choices
1 Starch   1/2 Fruit   1/2 Fat-Free Milk   1/2 Fat

Basic Nutritional Values

Calories	165
Calories from Fat	40
Total Fat	4.5 g
Saturated Fat	1.4 g
Trans Fat	0.0 g
Cholesterol	0 mg
Sodium	40 mg
Potassium	385 mg
Total Carbohydrate	27 g
Dietary Fiber	3 g
Sugars	11 g
Protein	7 g
Phosphorus	220 mg

Banana Split Breakfast Smoothie

SERVES 2

SERVING SIZE 1/2 smoothie

1 cup   plain, low-fat yogurt
1 cup   chopped strawberries
     1   medium banana, sliced
1 cup   crushed ice

1 Put everything into a blender and push the button and your breakfast is ready to go.

CHEF'S NOTES: Pair this with a piece of whole-wheat toast spread with 1 Tbsp of almond butter and you are off to a great start of an active day.

Exchanges/Food Choices
1 1/2 Fruit   1/2 Fat-Free Milk

Basic Nutritional Values

Calories	155
Calories from Fat	20
Total Fat	2.5 g
Saturated Fat	1.3 g
Trans Fat	0.0 g
Cholesterol	5 mg
Sodium	80 mg
Potassium	605 mg
Total Carbohydrate	29 g
Dietary Fiber	3 g
Sugars	19 g
Protein	7 g
Phosphorus	210 mg

Nuts about Pizza for Breakfast

SERVES 1   **SERVING SIZE** 1 "pizza"

1	whole-wheat English muffin
1 Tbsp	almond butter
½ cup	sliced strawberries
1½ tsp	shredded unsweetened coconut

1. Split and toast English muffin.

2. Spread each half with almond butter.

3. Top with sliced strawberries

4. Sprinkle with coconut.

CHEF'S NOTES: This is such an easy breakfast to prepare. If there are children in your home they will enjoy making this "pizza" and eating their creations.

Exchanges/Food Choices
2 Starch   1/2 Fruit   2 Fat

Basic Nutritional Values

Calories	280
Calories from Fat	110
Total Fat	12.0 g
Saturated Fat	2.5 g
Trans Fat	0.0 g
Cholesterol	0 mg
Sodium	315 mg
Potassium	400 mg
Total Carbohydrate	37 g
Dietary Fiber	8 g
Sugars	10 g
Protein	10 g
Phosphorus	295 mg

Chicken and the Egg Omelette

SERVES 6

SERVING SIZE 1/6th omelette

½   medium green pepper, chopped
½   medium onion, finely chopped
2 tsp   olive oil
1 cup   cubed cooked chicken breast
4   eggs
½ tsp   pepper
¼ tsp   paprika

1 Sauté peppers and onions in olive oil until tender.

2 Add the chicken, and cook until the edges start to curl.

3 Beat eggs, adding pepper and paprika. Pour the eggs over the chicken mixture and cook over low heat until the eggs set.

4 Serve immediately.

CHEF'S NOTES: This is a real wake-me-up meal. I love the smell of onions and peppers sizzling in the pan.

Exchanges/Food Choices
2 Lean Meat   1/2 Fat

Basic Nutritional Values

Calories	110
Calories from Fat	55
Total Fat	6.0 g
Saturated Fat	1.5 g
Trans Fat	0.0 g
Cholesterol	145 mg
Sodium	65 mg
Potassium	150 mg
Total Carbohydrate	2 g
Dietary Fiber	0 g
Sugars	1 g
Protein	12 g
Phosphorus	125 mg

Sweet and Smoky Baked Eggs

SERVES 4

SERVING SIZE 1 tomato half

2	large ripe beefsteak or heirloom tomatoes
1 tsp	ground pepper
1 tsp	cumin
4	medium eggs
2 tsp	grated reduced-fat Parmesan cheese

1 Preheat oven to 350°F.

2 Wash tomatoes and cut in half. Scoop out the pulp and seeds, leaving about a 1/2-inch rim of tomato.

3 Place cut-side up in a greased glass baking dish.

4 Sprinkle each tomato half with pepper and cumin. Break an egg into each tomato "shell." Sprinkle each egg with 1/2 tsp of the cheese.

5 Bake until the eggs are set, roughly 25 minutes.

CHEF'S NOTES: Your farmers market is a wonderful place to purchase heirloom tomatoes. While they may not be as perfect in appearance as some you might see in the supermarket produce section, they will be perfectly delicious. The sweetness of the tomatoes and the smoky tone of the cumin make this an interesting twist on baked eggs. Once in a while I substitute a bit of goat cheese for the Parmesan.

Exchanges/Food Choices
1 Vegetable   1 Medium-Fat Meat

Basic Nutritional Values

Calories	85
Calories from Fat	40
Total Fat	4.5 g
Saturated Fat	1.5 g
Trans Fat	0.0 g
Cholesterol	165 mg
Sodium	85 mg
Potassium	255 mg
Total Carbohydrate	4 g
Dietary Fiber	1 g
Sugars	2 g
Protein	7 g
Phosphorus	115 mg

Applesauce Pancakes

1 cup	quick-cooking oats (not instant)
¼ cup	whole-wheat flour or buckwheat flour
¼ cup	white flour
1 Tbsp	baking powder
2 tsp	ground cinnamon
1 cup	nonfat milk
3 Tbsp	sugar-free applesauce
4	egg whites, unbeaten

1. Combine all the dry ingredients in a bowl.

2. Combine all the wet ingredients in a separate bowl and add the dry ingredients to the wet ingredients. Mix until combined. Do not overmix or the pancakes will be tough.

3. Using a ladle, pour 1/4-cup portions of batter onto a greased skillet or griddle that has been preheated.

4. When the pancakes start to bubble, turn them over and cook until golden brown. Serve with additional unsweetened applesauce.

CHEF'S NOTES: If you make your own applesauce and add cinnamon to it, you can eliminate cinnamon from the pancake recipe. This is a hearty pancake that will get your day off to a great start and keep those hunger pains at bay. If you aren't feeding a crowd, freeze the extra pancakes and use them another day.

Exchanges/Food Choices
1 1/2 Starch   1/2 Fat

Basic Nutritional Values

Calories	140
Calories from Fat	15
Total Fat	1.5 g
Saturated Fat	0.2 g
Trans Fat	0.0 g
Cholesterol	0 mg
Sodium	285 mg
Potassium	220 mg
Total Carbohydrate	25 g
Dietary Fiber	3 g
Sugars	4 g
Protein	8 g
Phosphorus	420 mg

Savory Breakfast Egg Custard

SERVES 4   **SERVING SIZE** 1 custard cup

4	eggs
2½ cups	low-sodium chicken broth
1 tsp	rice vinegar
1 tsp	reduced-sodium soy sauce
	Toasted sesame oil (for preparing custard cups)
	Chopped green onions (for garnish)

1 Preheat oven to 420°F.

2 Beat eggs until blended (but not frothy), add the broth, rice wine, and soy sauce and blend well.

3 Pour into custard cups or ramekins that have been wiped with toasted sesame oil and cover with foil.

4 Place custard cups in a large baking dish filled with hot water halfway up the sides of the custard cups or ramekins.

5 Steam/bake until the custard is set, about 15 minutes, and garnish with chopped green onions. Can be served hot or cold.

CHEF'S NOTES: Whenever I can, I purchase eggs at the farmers market. Usually they have been collected early that morning. If you are lucky enough to have access to eggs fresh from the farm, you will love the difference. This is a very comforting dish, excellent for breakfast or a light supper.

Exchanges/Food Choices
1 Medium-Fat Meat

Basic Nutritional Values

Calories	85
Calories from Fat	45
Total Fat	5.0 g
Saturated Fat	1.7 g
Trans Fat	0.0 g
Cholesterol	190 mg
Sodium	170 mg
Potassium	190 mg
Total Carbohydrate	1 g
Dietary Fiber	0 g
Sugars	0 g
Protein	8 g
Phosphorus	120 mg

Breakfast Baked Apples

SERVES 4

SERVING SIZE 1 apple plus 1 Tbsp liquid

4	medium apples (use McIntosh, Rome, or Braeburn; not Red Delicious)
½ cup	water
1½ Tbsp	blue agave syrup
1 oz	chopped walnuts
1 oz	raisins
1 Tbsp	cinnamon
1 Tbsp	dried orange peel

1. Preheat oven to 350°F.

2. Core the apples and put them in an 8 × 8-inch glass baking pan. Pour the water into the bottom of the pan.

3. Combine syrup, walnuts, raisins, cinnamon, and orange peel. Spoon the mixture into the holes in the apples.

4. Bake until the apples are soft.

CHEF'S NOTES: When you visit your farmers market, ask for the best baking apples available. You can substitute dried cherries for the raisins in this recipe. If you choose dried cherries, make sure they do not have sugar added to them. Always use dried fruits sparingly; they are a concentrated source of sugar.

Exchanges/Food Choices
2 Fruit   1/2 Carbohydrate   1 Fat

Basic Nutritional Values

Calories	180
Calories from Fat	45
Total Fat	5.0 g
Saturated Fat	0.5 g
Trans Fat	0.0 g
Cholesterol	0 mg
Sodium	0 mg
Potassium	265 mg
Total Carbohydrate	36 g
Dietary Fiber	6 g
Sugars	26 g
Protein	2 g
Phosphorus	50 mg

Peach Melba Smoothie

SERVES 1   **SERVING SIZE** 1 smoothie

1	medium ripe peach
½ **cup**	raspberries
1 **cup**	unsweetened almond milk
¼ **tsp**	coconut oil
4	ice cubes

1 Peel, cut, and pit the peach. Cube and place in blender.

2 Add raspberries, milk, oil, and ice cubes.

3 Blend until smooth.

CHEF'S NOTES: A ripe and juicy peach will add sweetness to this smoothie. The raspberries add a contrasting tanginess and the almond milk adds another layer of flavor. This smoothie will keep you satisfied and energetic until lunchtime.

Exchanges/Food Choices
1 1/2 Fruit   1 Fat

Basic Nutritional Values

Calories	140
Calories from Fat	45
Total Fat	5.0 g
Saturated Fat	1.3 g
Trans Fat	0.0 g
Cholesterol	0 mg
Sodium	180 mg
Potassium	560 mg
Total Carbohydrate	23 g
Dietary Fiber	7 g
Sugars	15 g
Protein	3 g
Phosphorus	65 mg

Delish Deviled Eggs

SERVES 6

SERVING SIZE 2 stuffed egg halves

6	eggs
¼	large onion, grated
2 Tbsp	lemon juice
1 tsp	curry powder
½ tsp	ground white pepper
Dash	red pepper flakes
Dash	salt
	Olive oil, as needed
	Paprika (for garnish)

1 Place eggs in a pot of water. Bring to a boil. Remove from heat and cover. Let sit for 10 minutes. Run cold water over the eggs and peel.

2 Cut eggs in half lengthwise. Scoop 5 yolks into a small bowl; discard the remaining yolk. Mash yolks together with onion, lemon juice, and spices. If mixture is too dry, add olive oil 1 drop at a time until the mixture is creamy.

3 Stuff the mixture back into the hollows in the eggs.

4 Chill until ready to serve. Sprinkle eggs with paprika before serving.

CHEF'S NOTES: Deviled eggs for breakfast? Why not! If you prepare these the night before you will have a nutritious way to quickly start your day. I always buy two dozen eggs at my farmers market. One dozen to use that week and the other to hard boil for the next week. The fresher eggs are usually more difficult to peel.

Exchanges/Food Choices
1 Medium-Fat Meat

Basic Nutritional Values

Calories	70
Calories from Fat	35
Total Fat	4.0 g
Saturated Fat	1.3 g
Trans Fat	0.0 g
Cholesterol	155 mg
Sodium	70 mg
Potassium	90 mg
Total Carbohydrate	2 g
Dietary Fiber	0 g
Sugars	1 g
Protein	6 g
Phosphorus	90 mg

Tips and Guidelines for People with Diabetes

As people with diabetes, we need to make sure we SAVOR not only our food, but all the moments of our lives. Here's what the word SAVOR means to me:

S—Stop skipping meals
A—Avoid added sugar and salt
V—Variety of vegetables and fruits at every meal
O—Observe what's on the label
R—Regular exercise, regular testing, regular rest

These are some of the most important rules I have been following since I was diagnosed. I have always been a very energetic and on-the-go type of person. I had so many goals and wanted to get them all done. That is not a bad thing! But working like that without taking the needs of my body into account took its toll. I hope these guidelines will help you avoid a similar situation.

Stop skipping meals. Before my diagnosis I ate a lot of meals on the go. Often I skipped breakfast or grabbed a donut or some other sweet treat, thinking it would give me energy. Bad idea! Even when people who don't have diabetes eat this type of food they experience blood glucose spikes and drops. When we eat a healthy breakfast we give our bodies what they need to get started for the day. Your metabolism gets the kind of kick start it needs. Check out the variety of breakfast recipes I have for you. There are delicious selections for all tastes.

Avoid added sugar and salt. I have a friend who reaches for the salt shaker before he even reaches for his fork. As he shakes sodium all over his food I just shake my head. People with diabetes, and everyone else for that matter, need to be aware of the dangers of high blood pressure. We also need to retrain our taste buds. We need to learn to appreciate the true, naturally delicious flavors of the foods we eat.

Variety of vegetables and fruits at every meal. To succeed we should never do anything halfway. But, "half" is important when it comes to meal planning for people with diabetes. Half of our plates should be filled with vegetables and fruits. These foods provide soluble fiber, which helps slows down the absorption of carbohydrates and helps you feel full longer. Seasoning your vegetables with herbs and spices instead of rich sauces will help with weight control as well. Bananas (yes, bananas!), grapefruit, oranges, and apples are great choices for any meal or snack.

Observe what's on the label. You may not be able to judge a book by its cover, but you can judge foods by the information on their labels. Remember to always check food labels; you will be amazed at some of the additives that are hitchhiking onto our plates. The most interesting reading in the grocery store is not found in the checkout aisle. An important suggestion: use some of your farmers market veggies and herbs to make homemade versions of your favorite store-bought products. You'll get great flavor without any additives.

Regular exercise, regular testing, regular rest. Exercising for three hours one day a week is not the way to go. Look at exercise not as a chore but as a choice to live healthier. Start small with a brisk walk to start your morning. It will help with your circulation, which is especially important for people with diabetes. If you have to begin with just five minutes, that's OK. Add a few minutes every day. After a few weeks you will find yourself looking forward to this time. Have trouble with your feet and legs? Try water exercise! It will give you the opportunity to have an effective workout without putting too much stress on your joints.

Do not skip testing your blood glucose! What you don't know can and will hurt you. Discuss your testing schedule with your doctor and do not deviate from it. Yes, supplies can be expensive if you do not have insurance. Search the internet for the best prices.

Shakespeare referred to sleep as the "chief nourisher in life's feast." People with diabetes need to enjoy healthy helpings from that "feast." Our bodies need that time to rest and recuperate from a day of fighting this disease.

The Perfect Pantry

Good ingredients in your home equal good nutrition for you and your family. If unhealthy foods never make it through your door, then you won't have to worry about being tempted to eat something you know you shouldn't eat.

Diabetes supplies can be costly. That makes being as frugal as possible extremely important. The fresh produce you purchase at your farmers market needs to be cared for like the treasure it is. Bargains aren't bargains if they end up in the compost heap!

When storing fruits and vegetables, it is essential to know which ones will be bad neighbors and which will get along. Some kinds of produce, such as apples, apricots, honeydew, and cantaloupe, emit high levels of ethylene, which help in ripening. Others, such as plums, pears, and peaches, are very sensitive to that gas. And please, never refrigerate your tomatoes. Not only are they in the "sensitive" category, they lose much of their flavor when refrigerated. Look into the use of some of the special storage bags for produce. There are several brands available. These bags absorb the ethylene gas and help your fruits and veggies stay ready for your table. Later in this book I will talk about your local extension office and the wealth of information they have to offer. They will have great ideas to help you keep your produce fresh and ready to use.

When you return home after shopping at your farmers market, remember: "PS"—prep and store. For example, clean your carrots, celery, and jicama and cut them into sticks. Then place them into containers filled with water and you have easy-to-grab snacks. When boneless, skinless chicken breasts are on sale, I purchase several family packs and poach the breasts with onions and celery until cooked through. I package them, some whole and some cubed, and freeze them. I also freeze the broth to use in future recipes.

Have you ever heard the children's story "Stone Soup?" There are many different versions and I have been told that it is based on a real event. In the story a group of soldiers are camped near a small village. They have no food left and are hungry. Several of them go into town and ask if the people have anything to spare to feed them and their fellow soldiers. It is the end of a long period of war and there is little food left in the village. The men are turned away by every person they ask. They return to their campsite empty-handed.

Then one of the older soldiers starts a fire, fills a large cooking pot with water, and heads back to the nearby village. He asks the first person he meets to help him find a large stone. The soldier tells the villager that he was planning on making stone soup. "Stone soup?" asks the villager, "That cannot taste very good." The soldier assures him that it is delicious but explains that it would be even better with an onion added. The onion is supplied. And little by little the villagers add the small amounts of vegetables and herbs they have on hand. And everyone, soldiers and civilians alike, enjoy a hearty meal.

I find so many lessons in that story. Each of us has something to share. Together we can help nourish each other with words of encouragement or inspiration or by sharing stories of our triumphs and our challenges. If we work hard together we can make a difference in the world of diabetes and the world as a whole.

Enjoy the soups and stews in this chapter! I hope that they give you the nutrients and comfort you need to be happy, healthy, and productive.

Chicken Barley Stew

Summer Sour Cherry Soup

Curried Leek and Lentil Soup

Easy Seafood Stew

Grand Green Gazpacho

Mmmm Mushroom Soup

Jade Soup

Avocado Summer Soup

2, 2, 2 Good Gazpacho

Luscious Low-Carb Tortilla Soup

Asian-Style Vegetable Soup

Cold Squash and Buttermilk Soup

Tomato Mushroom Soup

Spicy Lentil and Sausage Stew

Cuban Black Bean Soup

Chicken Barley Stew

1 Tbsp	olive oil
6 cups	water or low-sodium chicken broth
2	medium onions, coarsely chopped
3	large carrots, scrubbed and cut into "coins"
8 oz	pearl barley, washed and picked over
2	(6-oz) cans tomato paste
1	(15-oz) can kidney beans, drained and rinsed
2	cloves garlic, minced
1 tsp	cumin
½ tsp	oregano
½ tsp	thyme
1 tsp	chili pepper
½ tsp	ground black pepper
Dash	kosher salt
Dash	dried red pepper flakes
2	(8-oz) boneless, skinless chicken breasts, cubed

1. Add the olive oil to the water or broth and bring to a boil in a large soup pot. Add the onions, carrots, and barley.

2. Cook, covered, on medium heat until the vegetables are soft and the barley is tender (35–45 minutes).

3. Add the tomato paste, kidney beans, garlic, and spices. Add the cubed chicken. Simmer until the chicken is heated through, about 5 minutes.

CHEF'S NOTES: This is a rich stew with complex flavors. I like to pull some of my homemade chicken broth and cubed chicken breast out of the freezer to make this even easier to prepare. The next day I usually enjoy a cup of this stew and a small salad for lunch.

Exchanges/Food Choices

2 Starch   3 Vegetable   1 Lean Meat

Basic Nutritional Values

Calories	290
Calories from Fat	35
Total Fat	4.0 g
Saturated Fat	0.8 g
Trans Fat	0.0 g
Cholesterol	35 mg
Sodium	460 mg
Potassium	910 mg
Total Carbohydrate	45 g
Dietary Fiber	10 g
Sugars	8 g
Protein	21 g
Phosphorus	260 mg

Summer Sour Cherry Soup

SERVES 6

2 pints sour cherries, washed and pitted
1 cup grape juice
1 cup water
1 stick cinnamon
1 whole clove (do not use powdered cloves)
2 Tbsp Splenda Sugar Blend
2 egg yolks
1 lemon, grated (rind only)

1. Combine the cherries with the grape juice, water, cinnamon stick, clove, and Splenda Sugar Blend and heat on medium until the cherries are soft.

2. Remove the cinnamon stick and clove.

3. Beat the 2 egg yolks with several Tbsp of the hot cherry mixture, then purée in a blender with 1 cup of the hot liquid and 1/2 cup of the cherries.

4. Add the puréed mixture back to the saucepan and stir in the grated lemon rind. Serve hot or cold.

CHEF'S NOTES: This soup is a sweet/tart change of pace. Add 1 Tbsp plain, nonfat yogurt with a sprinkle of nutmeg on top for a refreshing summer lunch. Served cold or warm, this soup is full of vitamins A and C and antioxidants.

Exchanges/Food Choices
1 1/2 Fruit

Basic Nutritional Values

Calories	95
Calories from Fat	15
Total Fat	1.5 g
Saturated Fat	0.6 g
Trans Fat	0.0 g
Cholesterol	60 mg
Sodium	10 mg
Potassium	180 mg
Total Carbohydrate	19 g
Dietary Fiber	1 g
Sugars	16 g
Protein	2 g
Phosphorus	35 mg

Curried Leek and Lentil Soup

SERVES 10

SERVING SIZE 1/2 cup

1	large onion, coarsely chopped
1 Tbsp	olive oil
3	fat carrots, sliced into "coins"
2	large leeks (white parts only)
5	cloves garlic, minced
1/4 tsp	ground ginger (or 1 Tbsp freshly grated ginger)
2 Tbsp	curry powder
1 tsp	cumin
1 cup	green lentils, rinsed
6 cups	water

1. In a large soup pot, sauté the onion in the olive oil over medium heat. Add the carrots.

2. Wash the leeks thoroughly to remove any grit. Chop the white parts and add them to the onions and carrots. Add the minced garlic.

3. Sauté until leeks are tender. (Carrots will still be slightly firm.) Add the spices and stir so the vegetables are evenly coated. Add the lentils and the water.

4. Cover the pot and bring to a boil. Reduce heat to low and simmer for 25–30 minutes until lentils are tender, stirring occasionally.

CHEF'S NOTES: Low in fat and calories and high in fiber, protein, and iron, lentils are extremely versatile. I use them in soups, stews, or vegetarian loaves or patties. The leeks add a milder, slightly sweeter oniony flavor to this soup. If you are not using this dish as a vegetarian option you could substitute low-sodium, nonfat chicken broth for some of the water.

Exchanges/Food Choices

1 Starch   1 Vegetable

Basic Nutritional Values

Calories	110
Calories from Fat	20
Total Fat	2.0 g
Saturated Fat	0.3 g
Trans Fat	0.0 g
Cholesterol	0 mg
Sodium	20 mg
Potassium	360 mg
Total Carbohydrate	19 g
Dietary Fiber	6 g
Sugars	4 g
Protein	6 g
Phosphorus	125 mg

Easy Seafood Stew

SERVES 6   **SERVING SIZE** 1/2 cup

1 Tbsp	olive oil
1 Tbsp	coconut oil
1	large onion, chopped
2	cloves garlic, minced
1	(15-oz) can no-added-salt tomato sauce
2 cups	water (or 1½ cups water plus an additional ½ cup of clam juice)
½ lb	mussels, scrubbed and debearded
1 lb	sea scallops
1 tsp	red pepper flakes
1 Tbsp	Italian seasoning
¼ cup	clam juice
1	bay leaf
½ tsp	salt
1½ lb	cod filets, cut into bite-size pieces

1. In a stockpot, combine the oils and sauté the onion and garlic until golden brown.

2. Combine the rest of the ingredients except for the fish. Simmer for 30 minutes before bringing to a boil.

3. Add the fish, lower the heat, and cover the pot. Continue simmering until the fish is done (about 7 minutes). Remove bay leaf before serving.

CHEF'S NOTES: Feel free to use a different combination of seafood in this recipe. Don't like mussels, add a little more cod or other firm white fish. Clam juice is available in small bottles. If you cannot find it ask your grocer. If you substitute clams for mussels, steam them and use the broth instead of the bottled clam juice. When using steamed clams, add them at the very end. Some farmers markets have stands run by fishmongers. You can depend on fresh seafood at those stands.

Exchanges/Food Choices
3 Vegetable   4 Lean Meat

Basic Nutritional Values

Calories	255
Calories from Fat	55
Total Fat	6.0 g
Saturated Fat	2.7 g
Trans Fat	0.0 g
Cholesterol	75 mg
Sodium	515 mg
Potassium	750 mg
Total Carbohydrate	14 g
Dietary Fiber	3 g
Sugars	5 g
Protein	36 g
Phosphorus	440 mg

Grand Green Gazpacho

3	medium (about 6 oz) yellow tomatoes, seeded and chopped
2	small cucumbers, peeled and diced
1	jalapeño pepper, chopped
½	large green pepper, seeded and diced
½	large onion, diced
	Juice of 1 lime
2	cloves garlic, minced
1	sprig cilantro, chopped
2 Tbsp	olive oil
1 tsp	ground white pepper
Dash	salt
4	pieces sourdough bread with crusts cut off (4 oz), cut into cubes
1½ cups	water

1. Purée all ingredients except bread and water in a food processor.

2. Add the bread cubes to the purée and let sit for 3 minutes. Purée again and add the water.

3. Store in a large, covered bowl overnight. Serve cold. Garnish with slices of lime or cucumber.

CHEF'S NOTES: It may be difficult to let this unusual gazpacho sit overnight before enjoying a serving, but it will be worth it. The flavors marry together to produce a zingy soup. Yellow tomatoes are not usually as high in acid as some red tomatoes. The sourdough bread adds a different thickening element.

Exchanges/Food Choices
1/2 Starch   2 Vegetable   1 Fat

Basic Nutritional Values

Calories	130	
Calories from Fat	45	
Total Fat	5.0	g
Saturated Fat	0.8	g
Trans Fat	0.0	g
Cholesterol	0	mg
Sodium	130	mg
Potassium	345	mg
Total Carbohydrate	19	g
Dietary Fiber	2	g
Sugars	5	g
Protein	4	g
Phosphorus	65	mg

Mmmm Mushroom Soup

SERVES 6

SERVING SIZE 1/2 cup

2 Tbsp	olive oil
1	small onion, chopped
1	medium carrot, diced
2 lb	fresh mushrooms
1 tsp	nutmeg
1	bay leaf
6 cups	low-sodium chicken stock
	Salt and pepper, to taste

1. Heat the olive oil in a soup pot and add the onions and carrots, cooking until they're soft but not brown.

2. Add the mushrooms, nutmeg, and bay leaf. Cook until the mushrooms are soft (about 5 minutes).

3. Add the chicken broth and cover.

4. Simmer for 30 minutes. Remove the bay leaf. Adjust seasonings to taste.

CHEF'S NOTES: I like to use a variety of mushrooms in this soup. Since the mushrooms at my farmers market are not prepackaged, I am able to get just the amount of each type that I want to use. I usually chop one type and thinly slice the other type I am using.

Exchanges/Food Choices
2 Vegetable   1 Fat

Basic Nutritional Values

Calories	100
Calories from Fat	45
Total Fat	5.0 g
Saturated Fat	1.0 g
Trans Fat	0.0 g
Cholesterol	5 mg
Sodium	100 mg
Potassium	715 mg
Total Carbohydrate	8 g
Dietary Fiber	2 g
Sugars	4 g
Protein	7 g
Phosphorus	165 mg

SOUPS AND STEWS   27

Jade Soup

SERVES 4

1   (12.3-oz) package firm tofu
1   (32-oz) carton low-sodium
    chicken broth
1   quart water
1   (1-inch) piece of gingerroot,
    peeled and grated (or 2 tsp
    powdered ginger)
2   large cloves garlic, minced
2 Tbsp   reduced-sodium soy sauce
3   large carrots, peeled and cut into
    medium-sized "coins"
3   green onions, chopped (both
    white and green parts)
20   spinach leaves (stems removed)
1 Tbsp   dark sesame oil
Dash   crushed red pepper flakes

1   Drain tofu in a colander, then cut into small dice.

2   Pour broth and water into a medium-size saucepan.

3   Add ginger, garlic, and soy sauce. Add the chopped carrots. Bring to a boil.

4   When carrots are crisp/tender (about 15 minutes), add the green onions, spinach leaves, and diced tofu. Reduce heat.

5   Stir in sesame oil and red pepper flakes. Simmer until tofu is heated through.

CHEF'S NOTES: So you are telling me you don't like tofu? I didn't think I did, either, until I tried it in this spicy soup. Give it a try, you might find it as satisfying as I did.

Exchanges/Food Choices
2 Vegetable   1 Medium-Fat Meat   1/2 Fat

Basic Nutritional Values

Calories	145
Calories from Fat	65
Total Fat	7.0 g
Saturated Fat	1.5 g
Trans Fat	0.0 g
Cholesterol	5 mg
Sodium	420 mg
Potassium	555 mg
Total Carbohydrate	10 g
Dietary Fiber	3 g
Sugars	4 g
Protein	11 g
Phosphorus	170 mg

Avocado Summer Soup

SERVES 8

1	small onion, finely chopped
1	clove garlic, minced
1 Tbsp	canola oil
2	large ripe Haas avocados
¼ cup	lime juice
2 Tbsp	sherry
1	(14-oz) can low-sodium chicken stock (or 1½ cups homemade chicken broth)
½ tsp	hot pepper sauce
2 Tbsp	chopped fresh cilantro
2 cups	low-fat milk
Dash	kosher salt

1. Sauté the onion and garlic in the oil until soft and fragrant. Set aside.

2. Peel and chop the avocado. Purée in a blender or food processor with the onion and garlic mixture, the lime juice, and the sherry.

3. Add chicken broth and hot sauce. Process until blended. Pour into a large serving bowl and add the chopped cilantro and milk. (Use more or less to achieve desired consistency.)

4. Add salt to taste and chill for 2–3 hours before serving.

5. Garnish with more chopped cilantro.

CHEF'S NOTES: Some people like to use 1 cup of low-fat milk and 1 cup of buttermilk in this soup. This makes the soup slightly thicker and tangy.

Exchanges/Food Choices
1/2 Carbohydrate   2 Fat

Basic Nutritional Values

Calories	125
Calories from Fat	80
Total Fat	9.0 g
Saturated Fat	1.5 g
Trans Fat	0.0 g
Cholesterol	5 mg
Sodium	50 mg
Potassium	380 mg
Total Carbohydrate	9 g
Dietary Fiber	3 g
Sugars	4 g
Protein	4 g
Phosphorus	95 mg

2, 2, 2 Good Gazpacho

SERVES 6   **SERVING SIZE** 1/2 cup

2 lb	ripe tomatoes
2	medium zucchini
2	large cucumbers, unpeeled (English or hothouse)
1	small purple onion
4	cloves garlic, peeled
1	large red bell pepper
1 Tbsp	balsamic vinegar
1 cup	vegetable juice
Dash	salt
Dash	pepper

1. In food processor finely chop the vegetables and garlic in batches. Place into a large glass bowl.

2. Add balsamic vinegar, vegetable juice, salt, and pepper. Chill for at least an hour.

CHEF'S NOTES: This will taste like summer even in October. Bring a bottle of your favorite hot sauce to the table so that those who, like me, enjoy a bit more spice can add some to their bowl.

Exchanges/Food Choices
4 Vegetable

Basic Nutritional Values

Calories	85	
Calories from Fat	5	
Total Fat	0.5	g
Saturated Fat	0.1	g
Trans Fat	0.0	g
Cholesterol	0	mg
Sodium	110	mg
Potassium	880	mg
Total Carbohydrate	19	g
Dietary Fiber	4	g
Sugars	11	g
Protein	4	g
Phosphorus	115	mg

Luscious Low-Carb Tortilla Soup

SERVES 6   **SERVING SIZE** 1/2 cup

2 (7-inch) low-carb, whole-wheat tortillas (such as La Tortilla Factory tortillas)

1 medium onion, chopped

2 (6-oz) boneless, skinless chicken breasts, coarsely chopped

4 large (4-oz) Roma tomatoes, peeled, seeded, and chopped

1 (7.75-oz) can diced jalapeños, drained and rinsed

3 (10.75-oz) cans low-sodium chicken broth

2 Tbsp cumin

2 tsp oregano

2 cloves garlic, minced

1 tsp chili powder

1. Preheat oven to 350°F.

2. Cut the tortillas into thin strips and bake until crisp. (Don't let them burn!)

3. In a skillet, sauté the onion and the chicken pieces.

4. Combine the tomatoes, diced jalapeños, chicken broth, and spices in a large saucepan. Add the sautéed chicken and onion.

5. Bring to a boil, then reduce heat and simmer, uncovered, for 40–45 minutes. Garnish with toasted tortilla pieces.

CHEF'S NOTES: Here, again, preplanning cuts down on preparation time. Grab one of those bags of poached, cubed chicken from your freezer the night before cooking this tortilla soup and it will be ready in record time.

Exchanges/Food Choices
2 Vegetable   2 Lean Meat   1/2 Fat

Basic Nutritional Values

Calories	165	
Calories from Fat	65	
Total Fat	7.0	g
Saturated Fat	1.2	g
Trans Fat	0.0	g
Cholesterol	35	mg
Sodium	380	mg
Potassium	480	mg
Total Carbohydrate	11	g
Dietary Fiber	4	g
Sugars	3	g
Protein	16	g
Phosphorus	155	mg

Asian-Style Vegetable Soup

SERVES 8   **SERVING SIZE** 1/2 cup

5 cups	chopped vegetables (bell pepper, asparagus, broccoli, carrots)
2 Tbsp	peanut oil
5 cups	low-sodium vegetable broth
1 cup	dry white wine (or add an additional cup vegetable broth)
1	medium onion, chopped
1 Tbsp	minced garlic (or 1 tsp garlic powder)
⅓ cup	grated fresh ginger
1	(14-oz) can light coconut milk
1½ Tbsp	fish sauce (nam pla)
3 Tbsp	reduced-sodium soy sauce
2 Tbsp	chopped fresh lemon grass
2–3	Thai chile peppers, chopped
1 cup	uncooked brown rice
1 cup	plain, nonfat yogurt (optional)

1. In a medium-size stock pot stir-fry the vegetables in the peanut oil for 5 minutes until they are crisp/tender.

2. Add all the rest of the ingredients except for the rice and yogurt.

3. Simmer for 25 minutes, stirring occasionally.

4. Cook rice according to package directions. Drain and add to the soup.

5. Serve as is, or stir in the yogurt to make the soup creamier.

CHEF'S NOTES: For a lower-carb version of this dish, you can substitute 1 (7-oz) package of rinsed and cut-up shirataki (yam thread) noodles for the brown rice. Simply cover the noodles with water and simmer for 10 minutes. Then drain the noodles and add them to the soup after it has simmered for 25 minutes.

Exchanges/Food Choices
1 1/2 Starch   2 Vegetable   1 1/2 Fat

Basic Nutritional Values

Calories	235
Calories from Fat	65
Total Fat	7.0 g
Saturated Fat	3.4 g
Trans Fat	0.0 g
Cholesterol	0 mg
Sodium	580 mg
Potassium	525 mg
Total Carbohydrate	35 g
Dietary Fiber	5 g
Sugars	6 g
Protein	6 g
Phosphorus	230 mg

Cold Squash and Buttermilk Soup

SERVES 4

SERVING SIZE 1/2 cup

1	small onion, diced
1 Tbsp	olive oil
1	quart low-sodium chicken broth
8	small yellow squash, thinly sliced
2 cups	low-fat (1%) buttermilk
1 Tbsp	minced fresh dill (or 1 tsp dried dill)
1 tsp	minced fresh chives
½ tsp	salt
½ tsp	ground black pepper

1. Sauté the onion in the olive oil until soft and golden in a large saucepan, then pour in the chicken broth.

2. Bring the broth to a boil, then add squash slices, cooking for 15 minutes.

3. Remove soup from heat and set aside to cool.

4. Process the soup in a blender or food processor until it's just slightly chunky.

5. Pour into large bowl and stir in the buttermilk, dill, chives, salt, and pepper. Cover and chill for an hour and serve cold.

CHEF'S NOTES: Buttermilk adds smoothness and a tart taste to this cold and refreshing soup. Try substituting small, young zucchini for the yellow squash or use half of each.

Exchanges/Food Choices
1/2 Fat-Free Milk   2 Vegetable   1 Fat

Basic Nutritional Values

Calories	145
Calories from Fat	45
Total Fat	5.0 g
Saturated Fat	1.4 g
Trans Fat	0.0 g
Cholesterol	10 mg
Sodium	505 mg
Potassium	1025 mg
Total Carbohydrate	17 g
Dietary Fiber	3 g
Sugars	12 g
Protein	10 g
Phosphorus	235 mg

Tomato Mushroom Soup

1	medium onion, chopped
1	clove garlic, minced
2 Tbsp	olive oil
5	large fresh or dried mushrooms, chopped
1	(14.5-oz) can stewed tomatoes, undrained
1	quart water
½ tsp	marjoram
½ tsp	ground black pepper
	Salt, to taste
Dash	Worcestershire sauce
1	small potato (Russet or Yukon), peeled and diced
½ cup	garbanzo beans
3 Tbsp	pearl barley

1 In a large saucepan, brown the onions and garlic in the olive oil until golden brown. Add the mushrooms and sauté for another 1–2 minutes.

2 Add the stewed tomatoes (juice and all) and stir. Cook for another 2 minutes or so.

3 Add 1 quart water and bring to a boil.

4 Add the marjoram, pepper, salt, Worcestershire sauce, diced potato, garbanzo beans, and the barley. Cover and reduce heat. Simmer on low heat for an hour.

CHEF'S NOTES: When I discover big, beautiful beefsteak tomatoes at my farmers market, I substitute them for the can of stewed tomatoes. I just chop up 2 large or 3 small tomatoes and 1 small green pepper and add them along with 2 minced cloves of garlic. If you do use a can of stewed tomatoes be sure to check labels and choose a brand that does not have added sugar.

Exchanges/Food Choices
1/2 Starch   2 Vegetable   1 Fat

Basic Nutritional Values

Calories	125
Calories from Fat	45
Total Fat	5.0 g
Saturated Fat	0.7 g
Trans Fat	0.0 g
Cholesterol	0 mg
Sodium	175 mg
Potassium	340 mg
Total Carbohydrate	17 g
Dietary Fiber	3 g
Sugars	5 g
Protein	3 g
Phosphorus	75 mg

Spicy Lentil and Sausage Stew

SERVES 8   **SERVING SIZE** 1/2 cup

1 lb	hot Italian turkey sausage
1 Tbsp	olive oil
2	leeks, washed, trimmed, and chopped
2	medium carrots, peeled and chopped
1	small onion, chopped
1	celery rib, very finely sliced
1	jalapeño pepper, seeded and diced
1 cup	lentils, picked over
2	cloves garlic, minced
½ tsp	dried thyme
½ tsp	ground black pepper
1	bay leaf
4 cups	low-sodium vegetable stock

1. Cut the sausage into 1-inch pieces and set aside.

2. Heat the olive oil in a large, heavy saucepan. Add the leeks, carrots, onions, celery, and jalapeño pepper and stir over medium heat until onions are soft, about 5 minutes. Add the lentils, spices, bay leaf, and 3 1/2 cups of the stock. Cover and bring to a boil.

3. Reduce heat and simmer on low until the lentils are soft (about 45–50 minutes).

4. Add the sausage pieces. If the stew is too thick, add the remaining vegetable stock, cover, and cook 10 more minutes until sausage is cooked through and lentils are very tender. Remove bay leaf before serving.

Exchanges/Food Choices
1 Starch   1 Vegetable   2 Lean Meat   1/2 Fat

Basic Nutritional Values

Calories	210	
Calories from Fat	65	
Total Fat	7.0	g
Saturated Fat	1.6	g
Trans Fat	0.2	g
Cholesterol	35	mg
Sodium	555	mg
Potassium	560	mg
Total Carbohydrate	22	g
Dietary Fiber	7	g
Sugars	5	g
Protein	16	g
Phosphorus	245	mg

CHEF'S NOTES: I like to add one more step that helps subtract even more fat from this low-fat stew. After cutting the sausage into small pieces I place them in a nonstick frying pan with several Tbsp of water. I cook them over medium heat for 5 minutes and drain. Your stew will still have all the flavor of the hot Italian sausage but fewer calories.

Cuban Black Bean Soup

SERVES 8

3 cups	dried black beans
10 cups	water, divided use
2	large onions, diced
4	cloves garlic, minced
2	jalapeño peppers, seeded and diced
1 Tbsp	cumin
1 tsp	ground black pepper
1 Tbsp	fresh lime juice
1 Tbsp	chopped cilantro
	Light sour cream (for garnish)

1. Sort beans, discarding stones and other debris. Cover beans with water in a large bowl. Cover bowl and soak beans overnight.

2. Rinse and drain beans.

3. Bring 1 cup water to a simmer in a large pot and add onions, garlic, and jalapeños. Continue to cook until the onions are translucent. Stir frequently.

4. Stir in the cumin, pepper, and then add the drained beans and the rest of the water. Bring to a boil and then lower heat. Simmer, uncovered, for 2 hours or until beans are tender.

5. Remove half of the soup and purée in a blender.

6. Return the soup purée to the pot, stir in lime juice and cilantro. Serve with a small dollop of light sour cream as a garnish or more chopped cilantro, if desired.

Exchanges/Food Choices
3 Starch   1 Lean Meat

Basic Nutritional Values

Calories	270
Calories from Fat	10
Total Fat	1.0 g
Saturated Fat	0.3 g
Trans Fat	0.0 g
Cholesterol	0 mg
Sodium	125 mg
Potassium	785 mg
Total Carbohydrate	50 g
Dietary Fiber	17 g
Sugars	7 g
Protein	17 g
Phosphorus	280 mg

CHEF'S NOTES: Black beans are rich in iron and minerals. They are known to lower cholesterol and to help regulate blood glucose. A bit of lime adds a note of freshness to their rich taste.

I am sure we all know people who are more concerned about what they put into their vehicle than what they put into their body. Only a certain grade of gasoline will do. They have to use a special kind of oil or a special additive. They do all these things because they want their car to run well and last long. And after making sure their car is purring they head right for the drive-through where they order greasy food and jumbo sugary drinks to stuff themselves with. Then they wonder why they are tired, grumpy, and sick.

I am an actor and I have to confess that, when I was making movies in California, I sometimes ate those meals. Fast food and a frantic lifestyle added up to a Charles who was ready to crash in the afternoon. When you are filming a movie there is a whole lot of hurry up and wait. You might start at dawn and can work until late at night. A lot of those hours are spent doing the same scene over and over. It can be frustrating and if you aren't at the top of your game you might get progressively worse instead of progressively better.

On the set there was always food available. Lunchtime offerings included a huge green salad surrounded by big bowls of bright orange shredded carrots, diagonally sliced bits of pale green celery, ruby red chunks of juicy tomatoes, matchstick-size slivers of crunchy jicama, and much more. The produce was so fresh and tasty that I asked one of the caterers where it came from. "The farmers market," was the reply.

I give those salads some of the credit for helping me give the quality of performance I did in the Emmy-nominated production of *The Summer of Ben Tyler* for Hallmark. They gave me the energy I needed to make it through long, hot summer days of filming. I couldn't have asked for better co-stars or a better crew. And I certainly couldn't have asked for better salads!

salads

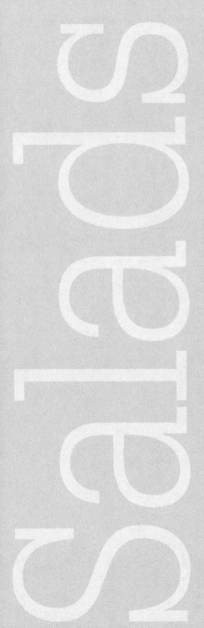
salads

Tabbouleh Salad

Berry Berry Good Spinach Salad

Chickpea, Tomato, and Cilantro Salad with Peanuts

Root Vegetable Salad

Shrimptastic Rice Salad

Tomato-Cucumber Salad with Lemon Juice

Bountiful Harvest Vegetable Salad

Crunchy Chopped Salad

Curried Four-Bean Salad

Veggie Barley Salad

Antioxidant Spinach Salad

Spicy Skinny Slaw

Mexican Tossed Salad with Avocado Vinaigrette

Waldorf Salad Skinny-Style

Bejeweled Spinach Salad

Chutney Chicken Salad

Cucumber Caprese Salad

Spicy Asian Vinaigrette

Tabbouleh Salad

SERVES 6

1 cup	bulgur (cracked wheat)
1 cup	cold water
¾ cup	minced parsley
2	green onions, chopped
½	medium green pepper, diced
¼ cup	fresh mint, chopped
1	large tomato, peeled and chopped
	Juice of ½ lemon
¼ cup	olive oil
	Salt and pepper, to taste

1. Soak bulgur in water for an hour, then drain well, pressing down with a spoon to get all the moisture out.

2. Mix bulgur with remaining ingredients. Add more lemon juice if needed.

3. Chill before serving.

CHEF'S NOTES: Nutty and chewy, bulgur wheat is an excellent complex carb for people with diabetes. Mixed with fresh vegetables and a tangy dressing, it is a satisfying side dish or main course.

Exchanges/Food Choices
1 1/2 Starch   1 1/2 Fat

Basic Nutritional Values

Calories	185
Calories from Fat	90
Total Fat	10.0 g
Saturated Fat	1.3 g
Trans Fat	0.0 g
Cholesterol	0 mg
Sodium	15 mg
Potassium	270 mg
Total Carbohydrate	23 g
Dietary Fiber	6 g
Sugars	1 g
Protein	4 g
Phosphorus	95 mg

Berry Berry Good Spinach Salad

3 cups	torn spinach leaves
¾ cup	sliced strawberries
¾ cup	blueberries
2 Tbsp	orange juice
½ Tbsp	olive oil
½ Tbsp	poppy seeds

1. Gently mix spinach and berries in a large bowl.

2. Stir together orange juice, olive oil, and poppy seeds. Toss lightly with spinach and berries.

CHEF'S NOTES: Often you will find spinach salads with high-calorie creamy dressings. But you can enjoy this version without guilt. Colorful and full of antioxidants, this salad is a powerhouse of nutrition.

Exchanges/Food Choices
1/2 Fruit   1/2 Fat

Basic Nutritional Values

Calories	55
Calories from Fat	20
Total Fat	2.5 g
Saturated Fat	0.3 g
Trans Fat	0.0 g
Cholesterol	0 mg
Sodium	20 mg
Potassium	215 mg
Total Carbohydrate	8 g
Dietary Fiber	2 g
Sugars	5 g
Protein	1 g
Phosphorus	30 mg

Chickpea, Tomato, and Cilantro Salad with Peanuts

SERVES 4

SERVING SIZE 1/4th recipe

3 cups	canned chickpeas, drained
½ cup	peanuts (raw or roasted, no or low-salt)
4	large tomatoes, chopped
1	green onion, chopped
1	small clove garlic, crushed
	Squeeze of lemon juice
	Few sprigs of fresh cilantro, chopped
	Drizzle of extra-virgin olive oil

1 Mix all ingredients together and drizzle with olive oil.

CHEF'S NOTES: Peanuts are related to chickpeas; they are both legumes. Peanuts offer more protein to your diet than actual nuts do. This salad gives you sweetness, crunch, and energy at a low price.

Exchanges/Food Choices
2 1/2 Starch   1 Vegetable   1 Lean Meat   2 Fat

Basic Nutritional Values

Calories	340
Calories from Fat	115
Total Fat	13.0 g
Saturated Fat	1.8 g
Trans Fat	0.0 g
Cholesterol	0 mg
Sodium	210 mg
Potassium	900 mg
Total Carbohydrate	43 g
Dietary Fiber	13 g
Sugars	12 g
Protein	16 g
Phosphorus	305 mg

Root Vegetable Salad

2   medium beets
2   medium turnips
4   large carrots
2   lemons
4   lettuce leaves

1 Wash and peel the vegetables.

2 Grate each vegetable into a large bowl, washing the grater between vegetables.

3 Squeeze the juice of the lemons over the grated vegetables and toss to coat.

4 Serve on lettuce leaves.

CHEF'S NOTES: Colorful, crunchy, and full of nutrients, this raw veggie salad has a natural, healthy sweetness that I find very satisfying. Give it a try. If you have any leftovers, add them to a stir-fry or soup.

Exchanges/Food Choices
3 Vegetable

Basic Nutritional Values

Calories	70
Calories from Fat	0
Total Fat	0.0 g
Saturated Fat	0.1 g
Trans Fat	0.0 g
Cholesterol	0 mg
Sodium	130 mg
Potassium	525 mg
Total Carbohydrate	17 g
Dietary Fiber	4 g
Sugars	9 g
Protein	2 g
Phosphorus	65 mg

Shrimptastic Rice Salad

SALAD

2 cups	cooked brown rice
1 lb	small cooked shrimp
1	medium green pepper, diced
1	celery rib, diced
1	green onion, sliced
1	(8-oz) can sliced water chestnuts, drained but not rinsed
	Salt and pepper, to taste

LEMON DRESSING

1 cup	plain, low-fat Greek-style yogurt
1½ Tbsp	lemon juice
2 tsp	prepared horseradish
1 tsp	grated lemon peel
½ tsp	salt-free lemon pepper
¼ cup	chopped cilantro (may substitute parsley)

1 Combine all salad ingredients.

2 Combine all dressing ingredients. Toss salad with dressing.

CHEF'S NOTES: Did you know that some people perceive cilantro as having a soapy taste? Researchers have determined that there is something in their physical makeup that causes this. If you fall into that category, by all means substitute parsley. If you use canned shrimp you should rinse and drain it before adding it to the salad.

Exchanges/Food Choices
1 Starch   1 Vegetable   2 Lean Meat

Basic Nutritional Values

Calories	160
Calories from Fat	20
Total Fat	2.0 g
Saturated Fat	0.7 g
Trans Fat	0.0 g
Cholesterol	120 mg
Sodium	590 mg
Potassium	255 mg
Total Carbohydrate	17 g
Dietary Fiber	2 g
Sugars	3 g
Protein	18 g
Phosphorus	265 mg

Tomato-Cucumber Salad with Lemon Juice

SERVES 4   **SERVING SIZE** 1/4th recipe

6 ripe large tomatoes, sliced into "rounds"
2 medium cucumbers, chopped into chunks
   Juice of 1–2 lemons
   Kosher salt, to taste
   Salt-free lemon pepper, to taste

1 Layer tomatoes and cucumbers in a large serving bowl, lightly sprinkling kosher salt and spraying lemon juice on each layer.

2 Top with a sprinkle of lemon pepper seasoning.

3 Refrigerate for at least 1 hour before serving.

CHEF'S NOTES: Here's a tip that will help save money and reduce waste—purchase some small plastic spray bottles at your local dollar store and put fresh lemon juice into one. When you need lemon juice just spray it on for the flavor you are looking for without leaving excess in the bottom of the serving bowl. Be sure to label the bottle!

Exchanges/Food Choices
3 Vegetable

Basic Nutritional Values

Calories	75
Calories from Fat	5
Total Fat	0.5 g
Saturated Fat	0.1 g
Trans Fat	0.0 g
Cholesterol	0 mg
Sodium	20 mg
Potassium	870 mg
Total Carbohydrate	17 g
Dietary Fiber	4 g
Sugars	10 g
Protein	3 g
Phosphorus	100 mg

Bountiful Harvest Vegetable Salad

SERVES 6   **SERVING SIZE** 1/6th recipe

1 Tbsp	hazelnut or olive oil
1	small onion, finely chopped
1	clove garlic, finely chopped
¾ cup	malt vinegar
1 Tbsp	brown sugar
1 cup	chopped parsnips
1 cup	chopped turnips
½ cup	parsley and cilantro leaves
8 cups	baby salad greens
½ cup	toasted walnut pieces
1 cup	chopped radish
	Salt and pepper, to taste

1 Heat oil in a large skillet over medium heat. Add onions and cook until golden brown, 5–7 minutes. Add garlic and cook for 30 seconds more. Stir in vinegar and sugar and bring just to a simmer. Remove from heat and keep dressing warm.

2 Bring a large pot of salted water to a boil. Add parsnips and turnips and simmer until vegetables are just tender, 8–10 minutes. Drain well.

3 Arrange parsley, cilantro, and salad greens and top with hot vegetables, then garnish with walnuts and radish. Drizzle with warm dressing, and serve immediately.

CHEF'S NOTES: This is a wonderful way to use fresh produce from first harvest to last. The contrast of the warm dressing, tender cooked veggies, and crunchy radish and walnuts over the salad greens is a treat for your taste buds. And this salad is full of nutrients for your body.

Exchanges/Food Choices
2 Vegetable   2 Fat

Basic Nutritional Values

Calories	145
Calories from Fat	80
Total Fat	9.0 g
Saturated Fat	0.8 g
Trans Fat	0.0 g
Cholesterol	0 mg
Sodium	45 mg
Potassium	415 mg
Total Carbohydrate	14 g
Dietary Fiber	4 g
Sugars	6 g
Protein	3 g
Phosphorus	85 mg

Crunchy Chopped Salad

6	Roma tomatoes, seeded and chopped
2	medium cucumbers (English or hothouse), peeled and diced
3	small radishes, very thinly sliced
½	small onion, chopped
½ cup	fresh mint, chopped
	Juice of 1 lemon
3 Tbsp	olive oil

1. Combine all ingredients and chill before serving.

CHEF'S NOTES: A quick and easy side salad. If Roma tomatoes are not in season, use 1 lb of grape tomatoes cut in half. I enjoy making this salad in the morning, then topping it with some water-packed tuna for lunch.

Exchanges/Food Choices
1 Vegetable   1 1/2 Fat

Basic Nutritional Values

Calories	85
Calories from Fat	65
Total Fat	7.0 g
Saturated Fat	1.0 g
Trans Fat	0.0 g
Cholesterol	0 mg
Sodium	10 mg
Potassium	270 mg
Total Carbohydrate	5 g
Dietary Fiber	2 g
Sugars	3 g
Protein	1 g
Phosphorus	35 mg

Curried Four-Bean Salad

1 Tbsp	olive oil
1 cup	balsamic vinegar
2	cloves garlic, minced
1 Tbsp	curry powder
1	(15-oz) can kidney beans, drained and rinsed
1	(15-oz) can garbanzo beans, drained and rinsed
1	(15-oz) can lima beans, drained and rinsed
2 cups	fresh green beans, blanched and cut into 1-inch pieces
½	medium purple onion, diced

1. Pour the olive oil into the bottom of a large bowl.

2. Add the balsamic vinegar, the garlic, and the curry powder. Whisk together.

3. Drain off the liquid in the beans and add them to the bowl. Add the diced purple onion. Using a slotted spoon, mix the beans, onions, and spiced oil and vinegar.

4. Refrigerate at least an hour, until ready to serve.

CHEF'S NOTES: Now, you just know I add a few dashes of hot sauce to this salad. I prefer to let it sit overnight for the beans to soak up all those good flavors. If your farmers market has fresh limas cook some up and use in place of the canned ones. When they are available, I substitute yellow beans for half of the green beans called for in this recipe.

Exchanges/Food Choices
2 Starch   1/2 Carbohydrate   1 Lean Meat

Basic Nutritional Values

Calories	250	
Calories from Fat	35	
Total Fat	4.0	g
Saturated Fat	0.5	g
Trans Fat	0.0	g
Cholesterol	0	mg
Sodium	300	mg
Potassium	650	mg
Total Carbohydrate	42	g
Dietary Fiber	11	g
Sugars	10	g
Protein	12	g
Phosphorus	205	mg

Veggie Barley Salad

1½ cups	low-fat, low-sodium chicken broth
1 cup	quick-cooking barley
1 cup	plus 1 Tbsp water, divided use
2	green onions, thinly chopped (white and green parts)
2	small plum tomatoes, seeded and diced
1	small green pepper, diced
1	summer squash, cut in half and sliced into half-moons
3 Tbsp	olive oil
3 Tbsp	apple cider vinegar
¼ tsp	salt
¼ tsp	ground pepper
¼ cup	roasted, hulled, unsalted sunflower seeds

1. Combine broth, barley, and 1 cup water and bring to a boil in a small saucepan. (Substitute vegetable broth for a vegan dish.) Reduce heat and cover, simmering until barley is tender, about 12 minutes. Set aside to cool.

2. Combine the vegetables in a large bowl. Stir in the cooled barley.

3. Mix the oil, vinegar, remaining 1 Tbsp water, salt, and pepper in a separate bowl.

4. Pour dressing over the barley and vegetables and chill for at least 4 hours.

5. Stir in the sunflower seeds just before serving.

CHEF'S NOTES: Barley is a wonderful source of soluble fiber and is considered a very good food for people with diabetes. It does contain some traces of gluten, so may not be appropriate for those who are sensitive to gluten.

Exchanges/Food Choices
2 Starch   1 Vegetable   2 1/2 Fat

Basic Nutritional Values

Calories	295
Calories from Fat	135
Total Fat	15.0 g
Saturated Fat	1.9 g
Trans Fat	0.0 g
Cholesterol	0 mg
Sodium	185 mg
Potassium	510 mg
Total Carbohydrate	35 g
Dietary Fiber	6 g
Sugars	3 g
Protein	7 g
Phosphorus	220 mg

Antioxidant Spinach Salad

SERVES 4

4   artichoke hearts (fresh, frozen, or packed in water), sliced in half
1   (10-oz) bag spinach leaves (or 1 large bunch spinach with stems removed)
1   large ripe avocado, diced
½ cup   unsalted sunflower seeds
1   small purple onion, diced

1   If using frozen artichoke hearts, defrost and drain before slicing and adding to the salad.

2   Combine all ingredients in a large salad bowl.

3   Toss with your favorite dressing.

CHEF'S NOTES: Be sure to rinse the spinach well. The avocado adds a richness to this salad and gives you lots of vitamin B6 and lutein. Lutein helps with eye health, which is of particular concern to people with diabetes.

Exchanges/Food Choices
1/2 Carbohydrate   1 Vegetable   3 Fat

Basic Nutritional Values

Calories	200
Calories from Fat	135
Total Fat	15.0 g
Saturated Fat	1.8 g
Trans Fat	0.0 g
Cholesterol	0 mg
Sodium	75 mg
Potassium	850 mg
Total Carbohydrate	15 g
Dietary Fiber	8 g
Sugars	2 g
Protein	7 g
Phosphorus	265 mg

Spicy Skinny Slaw

½   (12-oz) package broccoli slaw
¼   medium red cabbage, shredded
¼   medium green cabbage, shredded
1   large carrot, shredded
3   green onions, chopped (white parts only)

1 Combine ingredients in a salad bowl and dress with Spicy Asian Vinaigrette (page 56).

2 Garnish with a sprinkle of black sesame seeds (optional).

CHEF'S NOTES: You can find "broccoli slaw," which is just shredded broccoli stems, in your grocery store. But you can easily peel and shred your own. Buy a bunch of broccoli at your farmers market. Use the florets in one recipe and save the rest to use in this crunchy Asian salad.

Exchanges/Food Choices
2 Vegetable

Basic Nutritional Values

Calories	55
Calories from Fat	0
Total Fat	0.0 g
Saturated Fat	0.1 g
Trans Fat	0.0 g
Cholesterol	0 mg
Sodium	50 mg
Potassium	450 mg
Total Carbohydrate	12 g
Dietary Fiber	5 g
Sugars	6 g
Protein	3 g
Phosphorus	70 mg

Mexican Tossed Salad with Avocado Vinaigrette

SERVES 6   **SERVING SIZE** 1/6th recipe

SALAD

1	large head romaine lettuce
1	(15-oz) can garbanzo beans, drained and rinsed
1 cup	corn kernels (frozen or fresh)
1	large green pepper, cored and diced
1	small jicama, cut into french fry shapes
1 cup	cherry or teardrop tomatoes
1	small purple onion, diced
1	small bunch cilantro, chopped (optional)

AVOCADO VINAIGRETTE

1	large or 2 small Haas avocados
	Juice of 2 limes
1	clove garlic, minced
⅓ cup	olive oil
1 tsp	ground black pepper
½ tsp	cayenne pepper
Dash	dried red pepper flakes
Dash	kosher salt
	Water, as needed

1 Combine all salad ingredients and toss to distribute.

2 Whisk all Avocado Vinaigrette ingredients together to make a creamy dressing. Add to salad and serve immediately.

CHEF'S NOTES: If your local farmers market carries Fuerte avocados, a smooth-skinned green variety, substitute for the Haas avocados.

Exchanges/Food Choices
1 Starch   3 Vegetable   3 Fat

Basic Nutritional Values

Calories	300		
Calories from Fat	160	**Potassium**	770 mg
Total Fat	18.0 g	**Total Carbohydrate**	32 g
Saturated Fat	2.5 g	Dietary Fiber	12 g
Trans Fat	0.0 g	Sugars	7 g
Cholesterol	0 mg	**Protein**	7 g
Sodium	90 mg	**Phosphorus**	155 mg

Waldorf Salad Skinny-Style

SERVES 6

1 (6-oz) container plain, nonfat yogurt
1 Tbsp apple cider vinegar
1 large tart apple, coarsely chopped but not peeled
½ cup green seedless grapes, sliced in half
½ cup chopped celery
¾ cup chopped walnuts (unsalted)

1. Mix yogurt and vinegar together.

2. Add apple, grapes, and celery. Mix well.

3. Chill before serving.

4. Garnish with chopped walnuts.

CHEF'S NOTES: For a change of pace substitute 1/2 cup of chopped dates for the seedless grapes or add some cubed, cooked chicken breast and make this a light dinner.

Exchanges/Food Choices
1/2 Fruit   1/2 Carbohydrate   2 Fat

Basic Nutritional Values

Calories	140
Calories from Fat	90
Total Fat	10.0 g
Saturated Fat	1.0 g
Trans Fat	0.0 g
Cholesterol	0 mg
Sodium	25 mg
Potassium	215 mg
Total Carbohydrate	12 g
Dietary Fiber	2 g
Sugars	8 g
Protein	4 g
Phosphorus	105 mg

Bejeweled Spinach Salad

SERVES 5   **SERVING SIZE** 1/5th recipe

SALAD

2 cups   baby spinach leaves
½ cup   minced purple onion
½ cup   pomegranate "arils"
½ cup   chopped walnuts
½ cup   crumbled fat-free feta

VINAIGRETTE

1 Tbsp   balsamic vinegar
1 tsp   honey
1 Tbsp   olive oil

1   In a large salad bowl gently mix spinach, onion, pomegranate arils, walnuts, and feta.

2   Whisk together the vinaigrette ingredients and drizzle over salad.

CHEF'S NOTES: This a sweet and tart, colorful and quick salad. The recipe gives you an added benefit—a new word for crossword enthusiasts. A pomegranate "aril" is one of those ruby bubbles of juice and crunchy seed that are hidden inside the fruit. Containers of arils are available in some grocery stores and can be stored in your refrigerator for 2 weeks or frozen for a longer period of time.

Exchanges/Food Choices
1/2 Carbohydrate   2 Fat

Basic Nutritional Values

Calories	150	
Calories from Fat	100	
Total Fat	11.0	g
Saturated Fat	1.2	g
Trans Fat	0.0	g
Cholesterol	0	mg
Sodium	190	mg
Potassium	260	mg
Total Carbohydrate	10	g
Dietary Fiber	2	g
Sugars	5	g
Protein	6	g
Phosphorus	105	mg

Chutney Chicken Salad

½ cup	plain, low-fat Greek-style yogurt
2 Tbsp	mango chutney (Major Grey), finely chopped
2 tsp	curry powder
½ tsp	ground ginger
1 Tbsp	white wine vinegar
3 cups	chopped cooked chicken
4 cups	salad greens, roughly torn into bite-size pieces
1 cup	very thinly sliced celery
½ cup	golden raisins, plumped
¼	medium onion, diced
½ cup	roasted, no- or low-salt Spanish peanuts (optional)

1. Mix together yogurt, chutney, curry powder, ginger, and vinegar. Set dressing aside.

2. Combine the chicken and greens, celery, raisins, and onion in a separate bowl. Pour dressing over salad, tossing to mix in thoroughly.

3. Garnish with the Spanish peanuts if desired.

CHEF'S NOTES: Just a small amount of chutney adds such a lot of flavor. This main dish salad has many different tastes and textures. They add up to an absolutely delicious meal that is diabetes friendly.

Exchanges/Food Choices
1 Fruit   3 Lean Meat

Basic Nutritional Values

Calories	215
Calories from Fat	55
Total Fat	6.0 g
Saturated Fat	1.7 g
Trans Fat	0.0 g
Cholesterol	65 mg
Sodium	145 mg
Potassium	435 mg
Total Carbohydrate	17 g
Dietary Fiber	2 g
Sugars	12 g
Protein	23 g
Phosphorus	195 mg

Cucumber Caprese Salad

1 lb   Roma tomatoes, washed and cut into medium slices

1   medium English cucumber, cut into thin slices

3 oz   fresh mozzarella, cut into ¼-inch rounds
Cracked black pepper, to taste

4 tsp   olive oil

1   bunch (about 3 oz) fresh basil leaves (for garnish)

1 Top tomato slices with cucumber slices, then the cheese. Sprinkle with cracked black pepper. Note: Do not add salt to this recipe as the cheese is very salty.

2 Drizzle olive oil, about 1/2 tsp per serving, lightly over the caprese.

3 Garnish each "pile" with a basil leaf.

CHEF'S NOTES: English cucumbers are long and thinner than other "cukes." There is really no need to peel them. It is a matter of personal preference. Adding cucumber to the traditional caprese salad recipe adds a lot more fiber and makes this a more filling dish.

Exchanges/Food Choices
1 Vegetable   1 Fat

Basic Nutritional Values

Calories	65
Calories from Fat	40
Total Fat	4.5 g
Saturated Fat	1.5 g
Trans Fat	0.0 g
Cholesterol	5 mg
Sodium	60 mg
Potassium	240 mg
Total Carbohydrate	4 g
Dietary Fiber	1 g
Sugars	2 g
Protein	3 g
Phosphorus	70 mg

Spicy Asian Vinaigrette

SERVES 22   SERVING SIZE 1 Tbsp

1	clove garlic, minced
¾ cup	peanut oil
¼ cup	rice vinegar
¼ cup	water
2 Tbsp	reduced-sodium soy sauce
1 Tbsp	blue agave syrup (optional)
2 Tbsp	grated fresh gingerroot
½ Tbsp	chili oil (or more to taste)
Dash	red pepper flakes
Dash	salt

1 Combine all ingredients in a glass jar and shake to mix.

CHEF'S NOTES: This sweet and tangy dressing is great for salads. It is also a delicious marinade for chicken, pork, or fish.

Exchanges/Food Choices
1 1/2 Fat

Basic Nutritional Values

Calories	70
Calories from Fat	70
Total Fat	8.0 g
Saturated Fat	1.3 g
Trans Fat	0.0 g
Cholesterol	0 mg
Sodium	50 mg
Potassium	5 mg
Total Carbohydrate	0 g
Dietary Fiber	0 g
Sugars	0 g
Protein	0 g
Phosphorus	0 mg

Have you ever played that game that has rectangular-shaped pieces of wood that you stack up and then pull out one by one and place on top of the structure? Every move must be carefully made so that balance is maintained. The game ends when the stack of wood blocks sways and finally crashes down. You lose.

Maintaining balance is no game when it comes to meal planning for those of us with diabetes. We must plan carefully or we too will come crashing down.

The side dishes you find here can be great building blocks to use in your daily meal planning. Consider the big picture. Don't just plan a well-balanced lunch or dinner. Look at your day as a whole and include the proportions and components recommended by the ADA.

Although there are many fine main dishes later in this book, you can always make up a plate that consists of several side dishes. Keep the ADA's "Create Your Plate" system in mind: 50% of your plate should be non-starchy vegetables, 25% starchy foods, and 25% meat or meat substitutes. Add a piece of fruit and there you go! Having diabetes does not mean being hungry. It means being careful so you can be healthier.

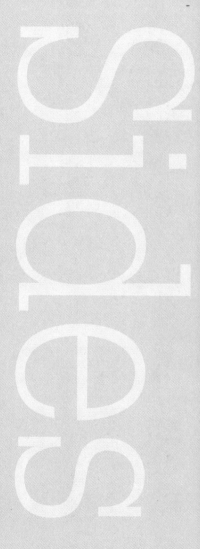

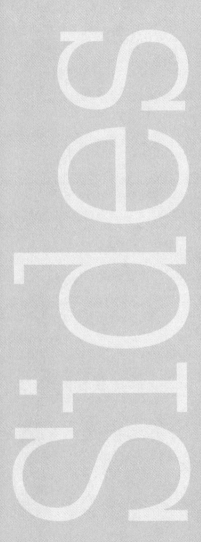

Sides

Jicama with Chile and Lime

Gingered Carrots

Rice Pilaf

Buckwheat with Lemon and Herbs

Armenian Eggplant Bake

Middle Eastern Lentils and Spinach

Vegetables à la Grecque

Rosy Rice

Asian Asparagus

Baked Polenta Italiano

Crispy Baked Broccoli

Cucumber Raita

Roasted Root Veggies

Chinese-Spiced Quinoa

Curried Confetti Rice

Stir-Fried Spicy Greens

Lemony Dill Pickles

Sunflower Soy "Butter"

Chinese Greens with Mustard

Chili Vegetable Summer Skillet

Vegetable Frittata

Stir-Fried Snow Peas

Basic Dal

Mediterranean Squash Medley

Roasted Brussels Sprouts

Tangy Green Beans

Herbed Batter Bread

Spiced Sweet Potato Fries

Roasted Asparagus with Garlic

Chickpea Crunch

Balsamic Veggie Bake

Hummus

Caribbean Cabbage Slaw

Jamaican Yam Curry

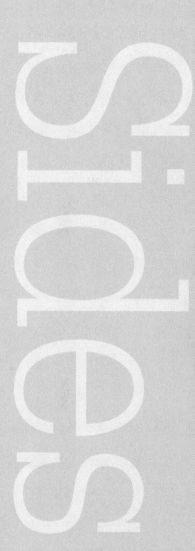

Sides

Jicama with Chile and Lime

SERVES 8

1 Tbsp	crushed red pepper flakes
	Juice of 2 limes
1	large jicama, peeled and cut into large matchsticks

1 Combine pepper flakes and lime juice in a Ziploc bag.

2 Add jicama pieces and toss to coat.

CHEF'S NOTES: Are you familiar with jicama? It resembles a turnip, is great raw, roasted, or sautéed, and has a mild sweet flavor. It is used quite a bit in Mexican cooking. When you are shopping for jicama steer away from the larger ones, they tend to be starchy. If you, like me, enjoy a bit more heat in your food, substitute a dried, crushed chipotle (a smoked jalapeño) or a tepin pepper for the red pepper flakes.

Exchanges/Food Choices
2 Vegetable

Basic Nutritional Values

Calories	60
Calories from Fat	0
Total Fat	0.0 g
Saturated Fat	0.0 g
Trans Fat	0.0 g
Cholesterol	0 mg
Sodium	10 mg
Potassium	240 mg
Total Carbohydrate	14 g
Dietary Fiber	7 g
Sugars	3 g
Protein	1 g
Phosphorus	30 mg

Gingered Carrots

SERVES 4   **SERVING SIZE** 1/4th recipe

1 lb	carrots, peeled and sliced into rounds
1 tsp	olive oil
2	cloves garlic, minced
1 tsp	minced ginger
½ tsp	nutmeg
1 Tbsp	lemon juice
¼ tsp	salt

1. Steam carrots.

2. Place oil, garlic, and ginger in nonstick sauté pan on medium heat and cook for 1 minute.

3. Remove from heat add carrots, nutmeg, lemon juice, and salt.

CHEF'S NOTES: Steaming is an excellent way to save time and nutrients. Ginger and lemon add heat and zing to this quick dish.

Exchanges/Food Choices
2 Vegetable

Basic Nutritional Values

Calories	55
Calories from Fat	15
Total Fat	1.5 g
Saturated Fat	0.3 g
Trans Fat	0.0 g
Cholesterol	0 mg
Sodium	215 mg
Potassium	335 mg
Total Carbohydrate	11 g
Dietary Fiber	3 g
Sugars	5 g
Protein	1 g
Phosphorus	40 mg

Rice Pilaf

1¾ cups	low-sodium vegetable or chicken broth
¾ cup	uncooked brown rice
2 Tbsp	olive oil
1 Tbsp	minced onion
1 Tbsp	minced garlic
1 cup	shredded carrot
1 cup	broccoli florets
3 Tbsp	minced fresh parsley
¼ tsp	salt

1 Bring broth to a boil. Add rice, cover tightly, and cook 35 minutes or until rice is done.

2 While rice is cooking add oil, onion, and garlic to nonstick sauté pan and cook until soft.

3 Steam carrots and broccoli.

4 When rice is done, add all ingredients together. Stir and cover. Let sit at least 15 minutes.

CHEF'S NOTES: If you have bits of leftover veggies in your fridge, add them to your pilaf. Add some cooked chicken breast and serve with a green salad for a complete meal.

Exchanges/Food Choices
2 Starch   1 Vegetable   1 Fat

Basic Nutritional Values

Calories	220
Calories from Fat	70
Total Fat	8.0 g
Saturated Fat	1.2 g
Trans Fat	0.0 g
Cholesterol	0 mg
Sodium	240 mg
Potassium	325 mg
Total Carbohydrate	33 g
Dietary Fiber	4 g
Sugars	3 g
Protein	4 g
Phosphorus	180 mg

Buckwheat with Lemon and Herbs

SERVES 5   **SERVING SIZE** 1/5th recipe

1 cup	organic untoasted buckwheat
1 Tbsp	olive oil
	Juice of 1 lemon, cut rind into long strands
5 Tbsp	minced flat-leaf parsley
4 Tbsp	minced chives
5	green onions, cut into shreds
	Salt and fresh ground black pepper, to taste

1 Rinse the buckwheat in a sieve under cold running water, put into a dry saucepan, and cook over a moderate heat for about 5 minutes, stirring from time to time, until it smells fragrantly toasted, and looks a bit golden.

2 Pour 2 cups boiling water into the saucepan with the buckwheat, standing back to avoid being scalded from the steam that may rise. Cover the pan, remove from the heat, and let stand for 15 minutes, or let stand over gentle heat if you want softer buckwheat.

3 Using a fork, stir the olive oil, lemon juice and rind, parsley, chives, and green onions into the buckwheat. Season with salt and pepper and serve.

CHEF'S NOTES: Buckwheat has a hearty, toasty, nutty taste. It is full of fiber and will give you lots of energy.

Exchanges/Food Choices
2 Starch

Basic Nutritional Values

Calories	150
Calories from Fat	35
Total Fat	4.0 g
Saturated Fat	0.6 g
Trans Fat	0.0 g
Cholesterol	0 mg
Sodium	5 mg
Potassium	225 mg
Total Carbohydrate	26 g
Dietary Fiber	4 g
Sugars	1 g
Protein	5 g
Phosphorus	125 mg

Middle Eastern Lentils and Spinach

SERVES 5   **SERVING SIZE** 1/5th recipe

1 Tbsp	olive oil
1	large onion, sliced
1 tsp	ground coriander
1 tsp	ground cumin
5 cups	spinach
2	(15-oz) cans green lentils, drained
1	clove garlic, minced
	Juice of ½ lemon
	Salt and pepper, to taste

1 Heat the olive oil in a large saucepan, add the onion, and cook gently for around 6–8 minutes, or until tender.

2 Add the coriander and cumin and stir for a few seconds over the heat as the aroma is released. Then add the spinach, continue to cook for around 10 minutes, as the spinach shrinks and becomes tender.

3 When the spinach is done, add the lentils and cook for a few minutes until they are hot. Then stir in the garlic, lemon juice, and salt and pepper to taste.

CHEF'S NOTES: The mouth-watering aroma of the spices will have you glad that this recipe comes together in very little time. Full of vitamin K, low in calories, and high in fiber, the ingredients in this recipe are known to be cholesterol reducers.

Exchanges/Food Choices
1 1/2 Starch   1 Vegetable   1 Lean Meat

Basic Nutritional Values

Calories	185
Calories from Fat	30
Total Fat	3.5 g
Saturated Fat	0.5 g
Trans Fat	0.0 g
Cholesterol	0 mg
Sodium	95 mg
Potassium	680 mg
Total Carbohydrate	29 g
Dietary Fiber	11 g
Sugars	4 g
Protein	12 g
Phosphorus	240 mg

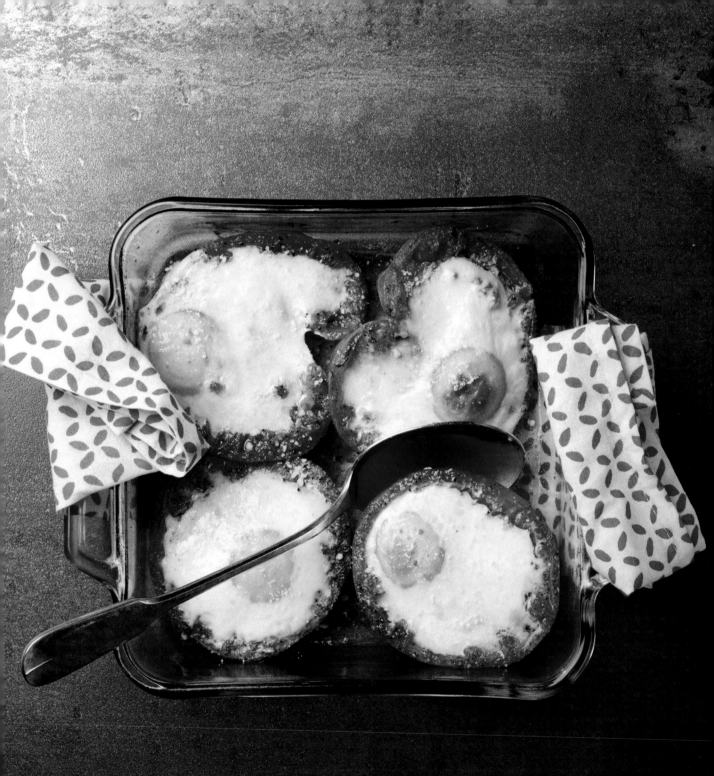

Sweet and Smoky Baked Eggs, page 10

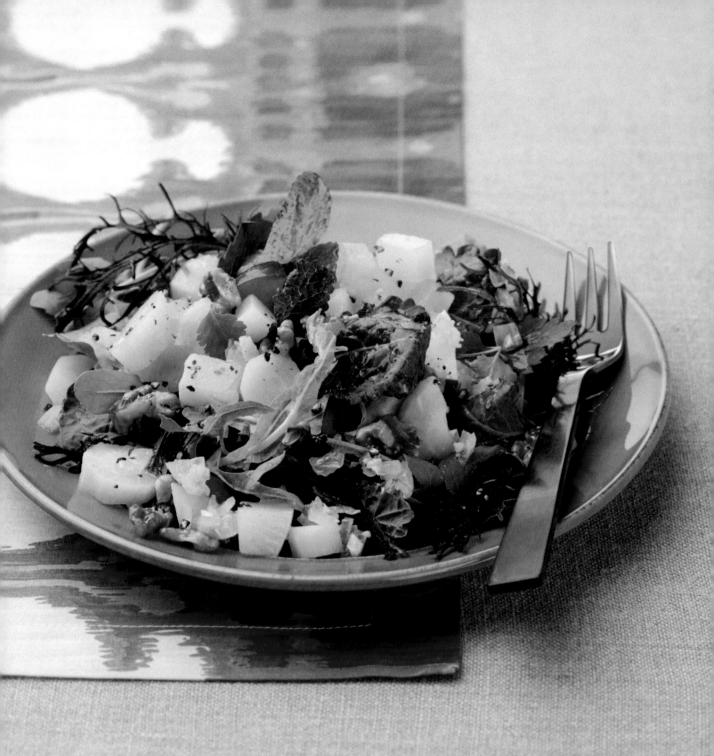

Bountiful Harvest Vegetable Salad, page 45

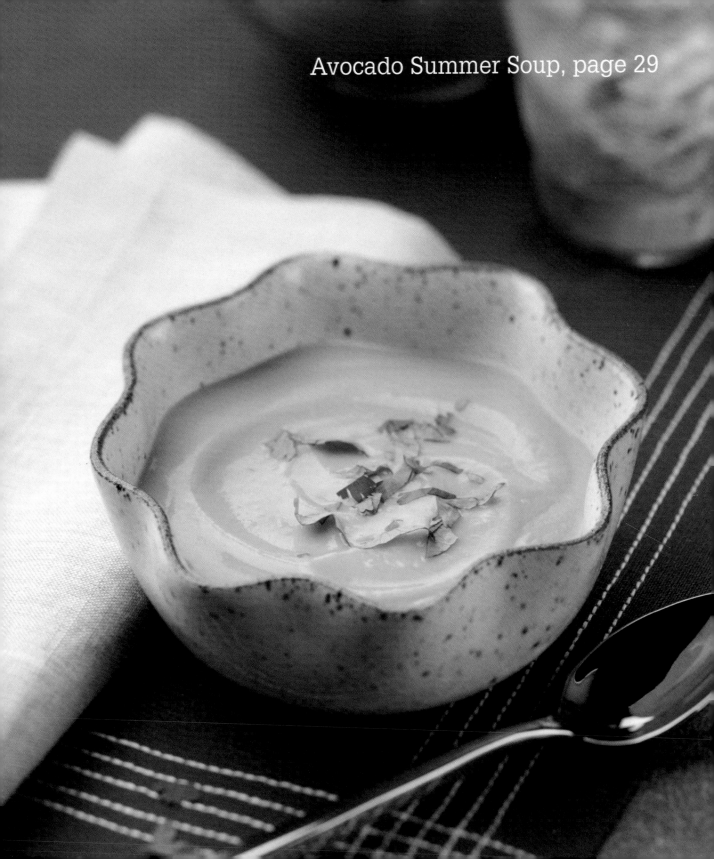

Avocado Summer Soup, page 29

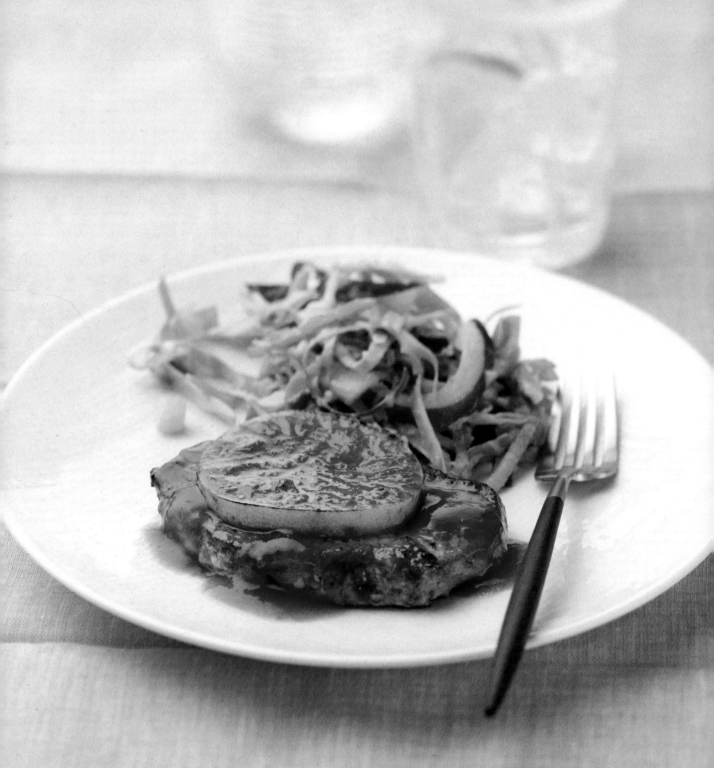

Citrus-Baked Pork Chops, page 100

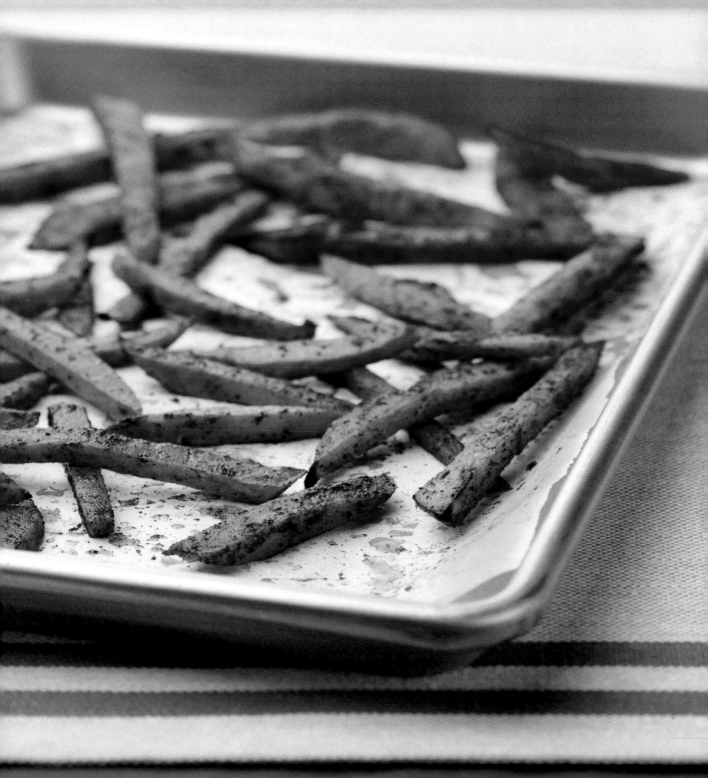

Spiced Sweet Potato Fries, page 86

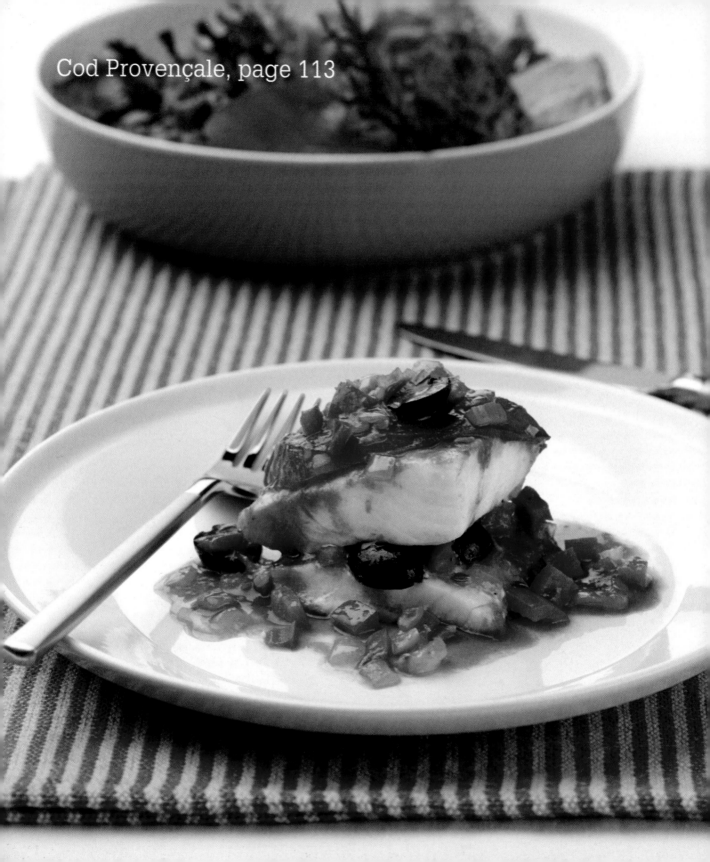
Cod Provençale, page 113

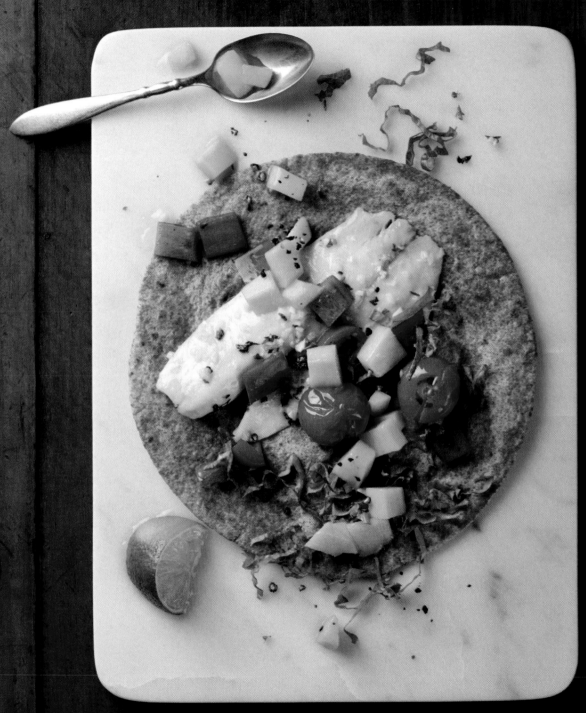

Fiesta Fish Tacos, page 114

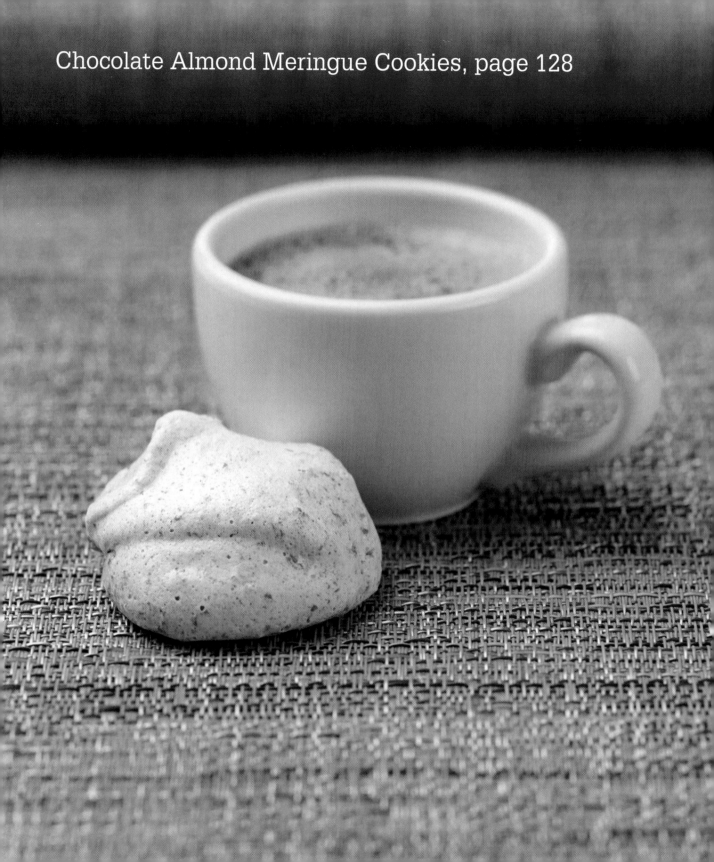

Chocolate Almond Meringue Cookies, page 128

Vegetables à la Grecque

SERVES 8

¼ **cup** plus 2 Tbsp olive oil, divided use
¼ **cup** white wine vinegar
½ **cup** water
½ **cup** dry white wine
½ **tsp** dried thyme
½ **tsp** oregano
½ **tsp** rosemary
½ **tsp** fennel seeds
½ **tsp** coriander seeds
½ **tsp** salt
  1 **lb** carrots, cut into matchsticks
  1 **lb** white mushrooms, chopped
  2 large onions, cut into thin wedges

1. In a large saucepan heat 1/4 cup olive oil, vinegar, water, and wine. Add the spices and salt. Bring mixture to a boil.

2. Stir in the carrots and reduce heat, simmering until the carrots are just getting soft (about 5 minutes).

3. Add the mushrooms and onions.

4. Cover and continue simmering until all the vegetables are crisp/tender (about 3 minutes). Remove from heat and stir in the remaining 2 Tbsp of olive oil.

5. Refrigerate for at least 2 hours before serving.

CHEF'S NOTES: There are lots of interesting spices in this dish. Spices and herbs can be your best friends. People with diabetes are not condemned to eating uninteresting meals.

Exchanges/Food Choices
2 Vegetable   2 Fat

Basic Nutritional Values

Calories	155
Calories from Fat	100
Total Fat	11.0 g
Saturated Fat	1.5 g
Trans Fat	0.0 g
Cholesterol	0 mg
Sodium	185 mg
Potassium	430 mg
Total Carbohydrate	12 g
Dietary Fiber	3 g
Sugars	6 g
Protein	3 g
Phosphorus	85 mg

Rosy Rice

SERVES 6

1½ **cups**	low-sodium chicken stock
1	small onion, diced
1 **Tbsp**	olive oil
2 **Tbsp**	marjoram
½ **tsp**	kosher salt
½ **tsp**	black pepper
½	(6-oz) can tomato paste
1 **cup**	uncooked brown rice

1. Bring the chicken stock to a boil in a large saucepan.

2. Sauté the onion in the olive oil in a skillet.

3. Add the onion to the boiling stock. Add the marjoram, salt, pepper, tomato paste, and rice.

4. Bring back to a boil, stir, then cover and immediately reduce heat. Simmer until the liquid has been absorbed, 15–20 minutes.

5. Remove from heat and let sit, covered, for 5 more minutes. Fluff with a fork before serving.

CHEF'S NOTES: The tomato paste adds an attractive color to this side dish. This rice pairs well with turkey meatballs. Or you can substitute vegetable stock or water for the chicken stock and make this a vegetarian dish.

Exchanges/Food Choices
1 1/2 Starch   1 Vegetable   1/2 Fat

Basic Nutritional Values

Calories	160
Calories from Fat	30
Total Fat	3.5 g
Saturated Fat	0.6 g
Trans Fat	0.0 g
Cholesterol	0 mg
Sodium	295 mg
Potassium	295 mg
Total Carbohydrate	29 g
Dietary Fiber	2 g
Sugars	3 g
Protein	4 g
Phosphorus	130 mg

Asian Asparagus

1	bunch thin asparagus stalks (about ²/₃ lb)
½ tsp	five-spice powder
1 Tbsp	reduced-sodium soy sauce
1 Tbsp	dark sesame oil
1 Tbsp	peanut oil

1. Trim the asparagus and cut off the tough ends.

2. Steam asparagus until crisp/tender, then set aside to cool.

3. Combine all the other ingredients except the peanut oil in a Ziploc bag. Add steamed asparagus pieces to bag and shake to coat with marinade.

4. Heat the peanut oil in a large skillet.

5. Add asparagus and marinade to skillet. Cook until asparagus is tender and the sauce is reduced and a little sticky. Stir often to keep asparagus from burning.

CHEF'S NOTES: Five-spice powder combines peppercorns, star anise, ground cinnamon, ground cloves, and ground fennel seeds. It is very powerful. A little goes a long way. If you like you can mix up your own to have on hand or purchase it already mixed.

Exchanges/Food Choices
1 1/2 Fat

Basic Nutritional Values

Calories	70
Calories from Fat	65
Total Fat	7.0 g
Saturated Fat	1.1 g
Trans Fat	0.0 g
Cholesterol	0 mg
Sodium	145 mg
Potassium	90 mg
Total Carbohydrate	2 g
Dietary Fiber	1 g
Sugars	1 g
Protein	1 g
Phosphorus	25 mg

Baked Polenta Italiano

SERVES 6

7 cups	water
1 tsp	salt
1²/₃ cups	coarse, stone-ground yellow cornmeal
1	large beefsteak tomato (or 2 Roma tomatoes), coarsely chopped
1 Tbsp	minced garlic
	Nonstick cooking spray
6	fresh basil leaves
2 Tbsp	grated fresh Parmesan cheese

1 Bring the water and salt to a boil and add the cornmeal slowly, stirring constantly.

2 Reduce the heat and continue to stir as the mixture thickens. When the polenta begins to pull away from the sides of the saucepan and is very thick (about 30–35 minutes), it's ready. Spread the polenta in a 1-inch-thick layer on a nonstick baking pan and allow it to cool completely.

3 Preheat oven to 400°F.

4 Combine the chopped tomatoes and the garlic.

5 Cut the cooled polenta into small (3 × 3-inch) squares, saving about 1/4 of the polenta for another meal. Spread the polenta pieces on a cookie sheet treated with nonstick cooking spray. Bake for 5 minutes.

6 Spread the tomato/garlic mixture evenly on top of the polenta squares. Top each square with a basil leaf. Sprinkle the cheese evenly across the polenta pieces and return to the oven.

7 Bake for another 10–12 minutes until the cheese has melted and the tomatoes are soft. Serve warm.

Exchanges/Food Choices
1 1/2 Starch

Basic Nutritional Values

Calories	105	
Calories from Fat	10	
Total Fat	1.0	g
Saturated Fat	0.3	g
Trans Fat	0.0	g
Cholesterol	0	mg
Sodium	325	mg
Potassium	155	mg
Total Carbohydrate	21	g
Dietary Fiber	2	g
Sugars	1	g
Protein	3	g
Phosphorus	75	mg

CHEF'S NOTES: I once heard someone say, "Polenta is just mush, trying to show off." As good as this dish tastes, it deserves to show off. You will build up some muscles making polenta; there is a lot of stirring involved. But it will be worth the effort.

Crispy Baked Broccoli

SERVES 4

Nonstick cooking spray
1 (16-oz) bag frozen broccoli florets
1 tsp garlic powder
½ tsp onion powder
1 Tbsp reduced-sodium soy sauce
1 Tbsp olive oil

1. Preheat oven to 375°F.

2. Prep cookie sheet with nonstick cooking spray.

3. Defrost broccoli and drain.

4. Combine remaining ingredients in a gallon-sized Ziploc bag. Add broccoli florets to the plastic bag and shake until coated.

5. Place florets on the prepared baking sheet with space between them. Discard leftover marinade.

6. Bake for 45 minutes to an hour. The broccoli will be soft inside but crisp at the edges.

CHEF'S NOTES: Check your broccoli after 30 minutes. Crispy can progress to too crunchy very quickly. This is an excellent way to serve broccoli to family members who are sure they don't like it.

Exchanges/Food Choices
1 Vegetable   1/2 Fat

Basic Nutritional Values

Calories	60
Calories from Fat	20
Total Fat	2.0 g
Saturated Fat	0.3 g
Trans Fat	0.0 g
Cholesterol	0 mg
Sodium	95 mg
Potassium	290 mg
Total Carbohydrate	6 g
Dietary Fiber	3 g
Sugars	3 g
Protein	2 g
Phosphorus	70 mg

Cucumber Raita

SERVES 6 (as an accompaniment to Indian or other spicy food)   **SERVING SIZE** 2 Tbsp

2 cups	plain, low-fat, Greek-style yogurt
1	medium cucumber, peeled and grated
2 Tbsp	chopped fresh cilantro
4 tsp	chopped fresh mint
1 tsp	kosher salt

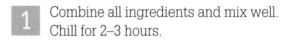 Combine all ingredients and mix well. Chill for 2–3 hours.

CHEF'S NOTES: This is a creamy, refreshing sauce. After you take a taste of something hot and spicy, raita will cool off your mouth so you will be ready for another bite.

Exchanges/Food Choices
1/2 Fat-Free Milk

Basic Nutritional Values

Calories	60
Calories from Fat	15
Total Fat	1.5 g
Saturated Fat	0.9 g
Trans Fat	0.0 g
Cholesterol	5 mg
Sodium	350 mg
Potassium	160 mg
Total Carbohydrate	4 g
Dietary Fiber	0 g
Sugars	4 g
Protein	8 g
Phosphorus	110 mg

Roasted Root Veggies

SERVES 4

Nonstick cooking spray
1 large purple onion, cut into wedges
4 large carrots, peeled and cut into chunks
2 parsnips (3½–4 oz each), scrubbed and cut into chunks
4 golden beets (about 4 oz each), trimmed and cut into chunks
2 Tbsp olive oil
12–15 cloves garlic, minced
½ tsp salt
1 tsp ground black pepper

1. Preheat oven to 425°F.

2. Prep cookie sheet with nonstick cooking spray.

3. The vegetable should be cut into pieces that are as uniform as possible so that everything cooks at the same rate. Combine the olive oil, garlic, salt, and pepper. Pour over vegetable pieces and stir to coat.

4. Arrange veggies on baking sheet with space between pieces.

5. Bake for an hour until the vegetables are soft and golden brown.

CHEF'S NOTES: Roasting brings out a natural sweetness in root vegetables that is pleasing and satisfying. If you can't find golden beets, red will certainly do.

Exchanges/Food Choices
1 Starch   3 Vegetable   1 1/2 Fat

Basic Nutritional Values

Calories	215
Calories from Fat	65
Total Fat	7.0 g
Saturated Fat	1.1 g
Trans Fat	0.0 g
Cholesterol	0 mg
Sodium	430 mg
Potassium	900 mg
Total Carbohydrate	35 g
Dietary Fiber	9 g
Sugars	15 g
Protein	4 g
Phosphorus	135 mg

Chinese-Spiced Quinoa

SERVES 4

2 cups	water
1 Tbsp	canola oil
1 tsp	Chinese five-spice powder
¼ tsp	ground ginger
¼ tsp	ground black pepper
1	cube vegetable bouillon (preferably no-salt)
1 cup	red quinoa, rinsed and drained (may use regular quinoa)

1 Combine all ingredients except quinoa in a saucepan and bring to a boil. Add the quinoa.

2 Reduce heat, cover, and cook until all the liquid has been absorbed, about 20 minutes.

CHEF'S NOTES: Eating red quinoa gives you a complete protein. Both regular quinoa and red quinoa have a nutty flavor, although the red is a bit more pronounced. The Chinese five-spice flavor helps make this an interesting dish that provides necessary amino acids.

Exchanges/Food Choices
2 Starch   1 Fat

Basic Nutritional Values

Calories	205
Calories from Fat	55
Total Fat	6.0 g
Saturated Fat	0.7 g
Trans Fat	0.0 g
Cholesterol	0 mg
Sodium	10 mg
Potassium	355 mg
Total Carbohydrate	31 g
Dietary Fiber	4 g
Sugars	3 g
Protein	6 g
Phosphorus	215 mg

Curried Confetti Rice

SERVES 6

SERVING SIZE 1/6th recipe

2 cups water
1 cup uncooked brown rice
1 (16-oz) bag frozen mixed veggies (corn, peas, carrots, and/or green beans)
½ cup unsalted sunflower seeds
2 Tbsp curry powder
1 tsp ground black pepper
1 clove garlic, minced
2 Tbsp olive oil
Dash salt

1 Bring the water to a rolling boil in a medium-sized saucepan.

2 Stir in the rice and add the rest of the ingredients.

3 Bring the water back to a boil, then lower heat, cover, and simmer for 45 minutes.

4 Turn off heat. Let sit, covered, for 45 minutes.

CHEF'S NOTES: The frozen mixed veggies I include in this recipe are not the ones you pick up from your freezer section in a grocery store. These are the ones you have purchased at your farmers market, frozen, and kept to be used in the winter months. Serve this with a large green salad mixed with assorted herbs.

Exchanges/Food Choices
2 Starch   1 Vegetable   2 Fat

Basic Nutritional Values

Calories	270
Calories from Fat	100
Total Fat	11.0 g
Saturated Fat	1.4 g
Trans Fat	0.0 g
Cholesterol	0 mg
Sodium	50 mg
Potassium	320 mg
Total Carbohydrate	38 g
Dietary Fiber	7 g
Sugars	3 g
Protein	7 g
Phosphorus	270 mg

Stir-Fried Spicy Greens

2 Tbsp	olive oil
¼	large onion, finely diced
1	Serrano chili, seeded and finely diced
2 lb	greens (spinach, collard greens, etc.), chopped and stems discarded

1. Warm oil in a heavy saucepan or wok.

2. Add onions, chili, and greens.

3. Sauté until the vegetables are tender, stirring frequently.

CHEF'S NOTES: If you choose spinach for this recipe it will cook down very quickly. If you choose collards or similar greens it will take longer. You can reduce the cooking time of those greens by rolling them up and cutting them in very thin strips. This is known as a chiffonade cut. Wash your hands well after cutting up that pepper and remember the seeds of a hot pepper contain the most heat.

Exchanges/Food Choices
2 Vegetable   1 1/2 Fat

Basic Nutritional Values

Calories	105
Calories from Fat	65
Total Fat	7.0 g
Saturated Fat	1.0 g
Trans Fat	0.0 g
Cholesterol	0 mg
Sodium	80 mg
Potassium	595 mg
Total Carbohydrate	8 g
Dietary Fiber	4 g
Sugars	1 g
Protein	4 g
Phosphorus	55 mg

Lemony Dill Pickles

SERVES 15   **SERVING SIZE** 2 slices

2	large (about 1 lb each) English cucumbers (or 6 Persian cucumbers)
2 Tbsp	kosher salt
1	clove garlic, crushed
2–3	stalks fresh dill
	Juice of 2 lemons, rinds reserved
2 cups	water

1 Thinly slice cucumbers. Place them into a bowl, and sprinkle them with salt.

2 Add garlic, dill, and lemon juice.

3 Grate the lemon rinds and add to the mix.

4 Add water and put all ingredients into a gallon-size Ziploc bag. Shake it up and marinate overnight.

CHEF'S NOTES: A few slices of these pickles alongside an open-faced sandwich or chopped up and scattered on a salad will add crunch and zing to your meal.

Exchanges/Food Choices
Free food

Basic Nutritional Values

Calories	10
Calories from Fat	0
Total Fat	0.0 g
Saturated Fat	0.0 g
Trans Fat	0.0 g
Cholesterol	0 mg
Sodium	465 mg
Potassium	95 mg
Total Carbohydrate	3 g
Dietary Fiber	0 g
Sugars	1 g
Protein	0 g
Phosphorus	15 mg

Sunflower Soy "Butter"

1 cup	roasted, salted soy nuts
1 cup	roasted, unsalted sunflower seeds
1 cup	dried cranberries
1 tsp	vanilla extract
1 Tbsp	cinnamon
1 tsp	grated fresh ginger
¼ tsp	kosher salt
1½ cups	cold water (more or less as needed)

1 Put soy nuts in a food processor and process until finely chopped.

2 Add the sunflower seeds and grind until fine.

3 Remove the soy nut/seed mixture and then grind the dried cranberries until fine.

4 Return nuts to the container with the cranberries. Add vanilla, cinnamon, ginger, and salt. Pulse to mix thoroughly.

5 Slowly add water until mix reaches spreadable consistency.

CHEF'S NOTES: This spread is high in protein and very high in flavor. It is nutty and tangy with sweet spice and the heat of ginger. Try this on a few low-carb crackers along with a bowl of soup.

Exchanges/Food Choices
1/2 Carbohydrate   1 Fat

Basic Nutritional Values

Calories	80
Calories from Fat	35
Total Fat	4.0 g
Saturated Fat	0.5 g
Trans Fat	0.0 g
Cholesterol	0 mg
Sodium	60 mg
Potassium	145 mg
Total Carbohydrate	8 g
Dietary Fiber	2 g
Sugars	4 g
Protein	4 g
Phosphorus	110 mg

Chinese Greens with Mustard

SERVES 6

SERVING SIZE 1/6th recipe

2 lb	bok choy (may substitute Napa cabbage or Swiss chard)
2 Tbsp	dry mustard
2 Tbsp	reduced-sodium soy sauce
2 tsp	rice vinegar

1. Bring a medium saucepan of water to a boil.

2. Clean and trim the bok choy, discarding any tough outer leaves. Cut the bok choy into slices. Add the sliced bok choy to the boiling water for 1 minute.

3. Drain and set aside to cool.

4. Combine mustard, soy sauce, and vinegar in a large bowl. Add the cooked bok choy and mix well.

5. Cover and chill thoroughly before serving.

CHEF'S NOTES: Bok choy is very high in Vitamin A, which is important in maintaining eye health. This is of particular importance to people with diabetes.

Exchanges/Food Choices
1 Vegetable

Basic Nutritional Values

Calories	30
Calories from Fat	10
Total Fat	1.0 g
Saturated Fat	0.0 g
Trans Fat	0.0 g
Cholesterol	0 mg
Sodium	270 mg
Potassium	355 mg
Total Carbohydrate	4 g
Dietary Fiber	2 g
Sugars	2 g
Protein	3 g
Phosphorus	65 mg

Chili Vegetable Summer Skillet

8	fresh jalapeño peppers (or 4 bell peppers)
1	small onion, diced
1 Tbsp	canola oil
4 cups	corn kernels (fresh or frozen)
4	large ripe tomatoes, seeded and chopped
½ tsp	cumin
½ tsp	oregano
½ cup	chopped cilantro or parsley
⅛ tsp	ground black pepper
Dash	kosher salt

1. Seed the peppers, then sear them over a gas burner until the skins blister and turn black. (If you don't have a gas stove, use the broiler.)

2. Remove the peels and chop the peppers.

3. Sauté the onion in the canola oil in a skillet until tender, then add the rest of the ingredients.

4. Mix well and continue to cook until the corn and tomatoes are a bit crisp. Can be served hot or cold.

CHEF'S NOTES: For those of you who may not be as fond of heat as I am, try a mixture of jalapeño and bell peppers. If your meal plan on the day you make this recipe already includes your allotment of carbs, feel free to substitute another, lower-carb vegetable for the corn. Zucchini goes very well in this dish.

Exchanges/Food Choices
1 Starch   3 Vegetable   1/2 Fat

Basic Nutritional Values

Calories	155	
Calories from Fat	30	
Total Fat	3.5	g
Saturated Fat	0.3	g
Trans Fat	0.0	g
Cholesterol	0	mg
Sodium	35	mg
Potassium	735	mg
Total Carbohydrate	31	g
Dietary Fiber	5	g
Sugars	9	g
Protein	5	g
Phosphorus	130	mg

Vegetable Frittata

SERVES 8   **SERVING SIZE** 1/8th recipe

	Nonstick cooking spray
2 Tbsp	olive oil
2	cloves garlic, minced
1	small onion, diced
1	medium zucchini, sliced very thin
4	large ripe tomatoes, seeded and chopped
1 cup	spinach leaves, chopped
½ cup	chopped fresh basil
½ cup	chopped fresh parsley
1	sprig fresh rosemary, chopped
12	egg whites
4 oz	fresh mozzarella, cut into cubes
	Fresh ground pepper, to taste
Dash	kosher salt

1. Preheat oven to 350°F.

2. Prep a large casserole dish with nonstick cooking spray.

3. Heat olive oil in heavy frying pan and add garlic and onion. Cook until onion is soft, stirring constantly.

4. Add the zucchini and sauté for another 1–2 minutes.

5. Add the chopped tomatoes and the spinach leaves, cooking for 2 minutes, then add the basil, parsley, and rosemary. Continue cooking until the herbs and spinach are wilted.

6. Combine egg whites, cooked vegetables, and the cheese in a bowl. Add salt and pepper if desired.

7. Pour the mixture into the casserole and bake for 40–45 minutes, or until the frittata is set. Cool before serving.

Exchanges/Food Choices
1 Vegetable   1 Lean Meat   1 Fat

Basic Nutritional Values

Calories	120
Calories from Fat	55
Total Fat	6.0 g
Saturated Fat	2.0 g
Trans Fat	0.0 g
Cholesterol	5 mg
Sodium	185 mg
Potassium	460 mg
Total Carbohydrate	7 g
Dietary Fiber	2 g
Sugars	4 g
Protein	10 g
Phosphorus	105 mg

CHEF'S NOTES: This is a great dish to serve to company. It serves 8 as a main dish, or more if you cut it into small cubes and use it as an appetizer. It is full of vitamins, minerals, and wonderful flavors.

Stir-Fried Snow Peas

SERVES 4   **SERVING SIZE** 1/4th recipe

2½ Tbsp canola oil
2 lb snow peas, trimmed
2 Tbsp tamari (or reduced-sodium soy sauce)
1 tsp toasted sesame oil
½ tsp garlic powder
¼ tsp Chinese five-spice powder

1 Heat canola oil in a heavy skillet or wok until it begins to smoke.

2 Stir-fry snow peas for 5 minutes. (They will be bright green with brown spots.)

3 Mix tamari with sesame oil and spices. Drizzle over hot snow peas and toss to coat before serving. Garnish with roasted sesame seeds if desired.

CHEF'S NOTES: Snow peas in your farmers market—a sure sign of the beginning of spring. If you do not usually cook with five-spice powder, please try it. It is sweet and spicy and adds a new dimension to stir-fry dishes.

Exchanges/Food Choices
3 Vegetable   2 Fat

Basic Nutritional Values

Calories	185
Calories from Fat	90
Total Fat	10.0 g
Saturated Fat	0.9 g
Trans Fat	0.0 g
Cholesterol	0 mg
Sodium	285 mg
Potassium	520 mg
Total Carbohydrate	16 g
Dietary Fiber	6 g
Sugars	9 g
Protein	8 g
Phosphorus	125 mg

Basic Dal

1 lb	dried split peas
5 cups	water
1 tsp	mild curry powder
¼ tsp	cumin
2 Tbsp	mustard seed
½ tsp	kosher salt
2	cloves garlic, minced
2	small onions, diced
4	large ripe tomatoes, peeled and chopped
¼ cup	canola oil
	Chopped cilantro (optional, for garnish)

1. Combine all the ingredients except the oil and cilantro and bring to a boil.

2. Reduce heat and simmer for 45 minutes, or until the peas are soft and the dal is thick and soupy.

3. Add the oil. Stir and simmer for another 15 minutes.

4. Garnish with chopped cilantro if desired.

CHEF'S NOTES: I enjoy the way peas are used in Indian cooking. They are extremely low in sodium and high in protein and iron.

Exchanges/Food Choices
2 Starch   1 Vegetable   1 Lean Meat   1 Fat

Basic Nutritional Values

Calories	270	
Calories from Fat	80	
Total Fat	9.0	g
Saturated Fat	0.7	g
Trans Fat	0.0	g
Cholesterol	0	mg
Sodium	130	mg
Potassium	805	mg
Total Carbohydrate	37	g
Dietary Fiber	14	g
Sugars	8	g
Protein	14	g
Phosphorus	195	mg

Mediterranean Squash Medley

3	medium yellow squash, sliced
3	medium zucchini, sliced
1	medium onion, diced
2 Tbsp	olive oil
3	beefsteak tomatoes, cut into slices
1 Tbsp	Italian seasoning
Dash	kosher salt
½ tsp	ground black pepper
1	clove garlic, minced

1 Sauté the squash, zucchini, and onions in the olive oil until they begin to soften.

2 Add the tomatoes, Italian seasoning, salt, pepper, and garlic. Simmer until the vegetables release their juices and are completely soft.

CHEF'S NOTES: If pattypan squash is available in your farmers market, try adding some of it in this dish. This type of squash is small and has scalloped edges. Add some whole when you add the tomatoes.

Exchanges/Food Choices
4 Vegetable   1 1/2 Fat

Basic Nutritional Values

Calories	150
Calories from Fat	70
Total Fat	8.0 g
Saturated Fat	1.1 g
Trans Fat	0.0 g
Cholesterol	0 mg
Sodium	55 mg
Potassium	1160 mg
Total Carbohydrate	20 g
Dietary Fiber	6 g
Sugars	11 g
Protein	5 g
Phosphorus	155 mg

Roasted Brussels Sprouts

SERVES 4

1 lb	fresh Brussels sprouts
2 Tbsp	olive oil
¾ tsp	kosher salt
½ tsp	ground pepper

1 Preheat oven to 400°F.

2 Trim Brussels sprouts and cut a little cross in the stem.

3 Blend oil with salt and pepper in a Ziploc bag. Add Brussels sprouts and shake until they're coated with the seasoned oil. Pour vegetables into a shallow baking dish.

4 Bake for 25–30 minutes, stirring and turning the vegetables every 5 minutes to prevent sticking and burning. (If it looks like the sprouts are going to burn, reduce the heat.) When ready to eat, the sprouts will be dark brown (nearly black).

5 Serve immediately or chill and serve as part of an antipasto platter.

Exchanges/Food Choices
2 Vegetable   1 1/2 Fat

Basic Nutritional Values

Calories	105
Calories from Fat	65
Total Fat	7.0 g
Saturated Fat	1.0 g
Trans Fat	0.0 g
Cholesterol	0 mg
Sodium	385 mg
Potassium	400 mg
Total Carbohydrate	9 g
Dietary Fiber	4 g
Sugars	2 g
Protein	3 g
Phosphorus	70 mg

CHEF'S NOTES: Try experimenting with different seasonings in the oil. The Chinese five-spice blend mentioned in an earlier recipe is delicious with the Brussels sprouts.

Tangy Green Beans

1 lb	fresh green beans
2	shallots, finely chopped
2 Tbsp	red wine vinegar
2 Tbsp	olive oil
1 tsp	dry mustard
1 tsp	cumin
½ tsp	ground black pepper
¼ tsp	kosher salt

1. Steam green beans until crisp/tender.

2. Drain and cool to room temperature.

3. Whisk together the remaining ingredients.

4. Pour dressing over green beans just before serving.

CHEF'S NOTES: I use my steamer almost every day. Such a great way to cook my veggies just the way I like them. The shallots add a mild onion flavor that enhances but does not overpower.

Exchanges/Food Choices
2 Vegetable   1 1/2 Fat

Basic Nutritional Values

Calories	110	
Calories from Fat	65	
Total Fat	7.0	g
Saturated Fat	1.0	g
Trans Fat	0.0	g
Cholesterol	0	mg
Sodium	125	mg
Potassium	195	mg
Total Carbohydrate	10	g
Dietary Fiber	4	g
Sugars	2	g
Protein	2	g
Phosphorus	40	mg

Herbed Batter Bread

SERVES 12

SERVING SIZE 1/12th recipe

1½ cups   low-fat cottage cheese
1 Tbsp   canola oil
1½ tsp   dry yeast
1½ Tbsp   honey
1 Tbsp   dry minced onion
1 tsp   garlic powder
1 Tbsp   Italian seasoning
1   egg
1 cup   white flour
1 cup   whole-wheat flour
¼ cup   wheat germ
    Nonstick cooking spray

1 Preheat oven to 350°F.

2 Combine the cottage cheese and oil in a large saucepan and heat through. Add the yeast, honey, onion, garlic, and Italian seasoning. Add the egg and beat everything until it is smooth.

3 Mix the white and whole-wheat flours in a bowl. Mix 1 cup of the flour mixture into the cottage cheese mixture. (If using a mixer, mix for 2 minutes; by hand, mix for 5 minutes.) Add the wheat germ and beat for another minute by hand. Add another 1/2 cup of the flour to the mix and beat for another minute. Add the last of the flour and mix using hands.

4 Cover dough with a clean towel and put in a warm place for the dough to rise. It will double in size in about an hour.

5 Punch the risen dough down. Prep a heavy 1 1/2-quart casserole dish with nonstick cooking spray and spread the batter evenly, as if making cornbread. Cover the dish and return the dough to a warm place but don't let it rise past the top of the casserole/baking dish.

6 Bake for 40–45 minutes. Invert on a platter and serve immediately, pulling pieces from the "loaf" as slices will fall apart.

CHEF'S NOTES: I encourage you to mix this by hand! If you have children, have them help. They will love it and you will encourage them to become involved in preparing the foods that will help them stay healthy. Years ago I might have planned my dinner and then just added bread or rolls without figuring them into the carb count. No more! This bread is a good accompaniment to a bowl of hot soup or a crisp salad.

Exchanges/Food Choices
1 1/2 Starch   1/2 Fat

Basic Nutritional Values

Calories	130
Calories from Fat	20
Total Fat	2.5 g
Saturated Fat	0.5 g
Trans Fat	0.0 g
Cholesterol	15 mg
Sodium	120 mg
Potassium	125 mg
Total Carbohydrate	20 g
Dietary Fiber	2 g
Sugars	3 g
Protein	7 g
Phosphorus	125 mg

Spiced Sweet Potato Fries

SERVES 6

Nonstick cooking spray
4 medium sweet potatoes (about 1½ lb total), washed and peeled
1 Tbsp olive oil
1 Tbsp ground cinnamon
1 Tbsp chili powder
½ tsp ground ginger

1 Preheat oven to 425°F.

2 Spray baking sheet with nonstick cooking spray.

3 Cut sweet potatoes into thick strips or wedges and put in a gallon-size Ziploc bag.

4 Add the olive oil and shake until the sweet potato pieces are coated. Place the uncooked "fries" on the prepared baking sheet in a single layer.

5 Mix the spices in a small bowl. Sprinkle the spice mix over the sweet potatoes.

6 Bake for 45 minutes to an hour.

CHEF'S NOTES: Sweet potatoes are a great source of vitamin A. They are lower than white potatoes on the glycemic index. These fries work well as a side dish with a main dish at dinner or as a side with a salad.

Exchanges/Food Choices
1 Starch   1/2 Fat

Basic Nutritional Values

Calories	90
Calories from Fat	20
Total Fat	2.5 g
Saturated Fat	0.4 g
Trans Fat	0.0 g
Cholesterol	0 mg
Sodium	40 mg
Potassium	370 mg
Total Carbohydrate	16 g
Dietary Fiber	3 g
Sugars	5 g
Protein	2 g
Phosphorus	45 mg

Roasted Asparagus with Garlic

SERVES 6

12	cloves garlic, leave whole
2 Tbsp	fresh thyme, chopped (or 2 tsp dried thyme)
2 Tbsp	olive oil
1/4 **cup**	water or low-sodium broth
1	bunch thin asparagus spears (1/2–3/4 lb), trimmed

1. Preheat the oven to 350°F.

2. Combine garlic, thyme, oil, and water or broth in a small bowl.

3. Divide asparagus into 6 servings and place on 6 pieces of foil large enough to wrap the vegetables into packets. Distribute the oil/herb/garlic mixture evenly over the asparagus and then seal the foil packages.

4. Place the foil packages on a baking sheet and roast until the asparagus is crisp/tender (about 20–25 minutes).

5. To serve, carefully unwrap the packages and slide the vegetables on a plate, pouring the juices on top.

CHEF'S NOTES: One of my beliefs is that there is no such thing as "too much garlic." If you prepare this dish when you are grilling, just place the packets on your grill and you will have little bundles of goodness to serve with your grilled chicken breast or whatever you choose to make.

Exchanges/Food Choices
1 Vegetable   1 Fat

Basic Nutritional Values

Calories	55
Calories from Fat	40
Total Fat	4.5 g
Saturated Fat	0.6 g
Trans Fat	0.0 g
Cholesterol	0 mg
Sodium	0 mg
Potassium	85 mg
Total Carbohydrate	3 g
Dietary Fiber	1 g
Sugars	0 g
Protein	1 g
Phosphorus	25 mg

Chickpea Crunch

2	(15-oz) cans of chickpeas
2 Tbsp	olive oil
1 tsp	cayenne pepper
1 tsp	ground ginger
1 tsp	ground cumin
½ tsp	salt
	Juice of ½ lemon

1. Drain and rinse the chickpeas.

2. In a big bowl, mix chickpeas with all the other ingredients.

3. Place on a cookie sheet and bake until nice and crispy. This should take about 30–45 minutes. Stir every 10 minutes.

CHEF'S NOTES: In the Caribbean you can buy fried channa (chickpeas) from street vendors. It's warm and crunchy and so delicious. Each vendor uses their own blend of spices but all are mouth-watering and nutritious. This baked version has much less fat but all the goodness.

Exchanges/Food Choices
1 1/2 Starch   1 1/2 Fat

Basic Nutritional Values

Calories	180	
Calories from Fat	65	
Total Fat	7.0	g
Saturated Fat	0.9	g
Trans Fat	0.0	g
Cholesterol	0	mg
Sodium	340	mg
Potassium	260	mg
Total Carbohydrate	23	g
Dietary Fiber	6	g
Sugars	4	g
Protein	7	g
Phosphorus	140	mg

Balsamic Veggie Bake

2	large purple onions
2	large eggplant
2	large sweet potatoes, peeled
4	medium zucchini
3	beefsteak tomatoes
¼ cup	olive oil
2 Tbsp	balsamic vinegar

1. Slice all vegetables into 1/2-inch slices.

2. Place vegetables in a 9 × 13-inch baking dish, with the tomato slices on top.

3. Whisk together oil and balsamic vinegar and drizzle over the top.

4. Bake at 300°F for 90 minutes.

CHEF'S NOTES: No spices or herbs on this one. You will taste the pure flavors of these fresh from the farmers market vegetables enhanced by a little balsamic vinegar.

Exchanges/Food Choices
1/2 Starch   3 Vegetable   1 Fat

Basic Nutritional Values

Calories	145
Calories from Fat	45
Total Fat	5.0 g
Saturated Fat	0.7 g
Trans Fat	0.0 g
Cholesterol	0 mg
Sodium	25 mg
Potassium	620 mg
Total Carbohydrate	24 g
Dietary Fiber	6 g
Sugars	10 g
Protein	3 g
Phosphorus	85 mg

Hummus

2	(15-oz) cans garbanzo beans, drained and rinsed
	Juice of 2 lemons
2	cloves garlic, crushed
2 Tbsp	tahini
½ tsp	kosher salt
½ tsp	ground black pepper

1 Combine all ingredients in a food processor container fixed with a metal blade. Hit purée.

2 Process until the mixture is creamy but thick enough to be scooped up with bread, crackers, or vegetables (about 1 minute).

3 Refrigerate if not using immediately. Serve at room temperature.

CHEF'S NOTES: If you don't have a food processor, microwave the garbanzo beans for 30 seconds, drain, and then mash with a fork before adding other ingredients. The resulting hummus will be chunky and less creamy.

OPTIONAL ADD-INS:
- Roasted bell peppers
- Roasted hot peppers
- Grated Parmesan cheese

I like a more chunky-style hummus, so I always mash the garbanzo beans rather than using a food processor. Although I mention the use of bread or crackers with hummus, I suggest using fresh vegetables from your farmers market to keep this more diabetes friendly.

Exchanges/Food Choices
1 Starch   1/2 Fat

Basic Nutritional Values

Calories	100
Calories from Fat	25
Total Fat	3.0 g
Saturated Fat	0.4 g
Trans Fat	0.0 g
Cholesterol	0 mg
Sodium	190 mg
Potassium	170 mg
Total Carbohydrate	15 g
Dietary Fiber	4 g
Sugars	3 g
Protein	5 g
Phosphorus	105 mg

Caribbean Cabbage Slaw

SERVES 10   **SERVING SIZE** 1/10th recipe

1 cup	plain, nonfat yogurt (not Greek-style)
1 tsp	blue agave syrup
2 Tbsp	apple cider vinegar
1	(6-oz) can crushed pineapple, drained
1	small mango, peeled and diced
1	Scotch bonnet pepper, seeded and minced (can substitute jalapeño pepper)
1	large purple onion, very thinly sliced
2	large carrots, peeled and grated
1	medium head green cabbage, shredded

1 Mix together the yogurt, agave syrup, and vinegar.

2 Add the pineapple and mango. Then add peppers, onion, carrots, and cabbage.

3 Mix well and chill before serving. Serve using a slotted spoon to drain.

CHEF'S NOTES: By draining the excess liquid off the slaw you reduce the calories. The cabbage will have absorbed all the flavors by then. Make sure your crushed pineapple does not have added sugar. Your body does not need it and neither do your taste buds.

Exchanges/Food Choices
1/2 Fruit   2 Vegetable

Basic Nutritional Values

Calories	70
Calories from Fat	0
Total Fat	0.0 g
Saturated Fat	0.1 g
Trans Fat	0.0 g
Cholesterol	0 mg
Sodium	40 mg
Potassium	340 mg
Total Carbohydrate	16 g
Dietary Fiber	4 g
Sugars	11 g
Protein	3 g
Phosphorus	70 mg

Jamaican Yam Curry

2 lb	yams or sweet potatoes
1	medium onion, chopped
2 Tbsp	olive oil
1 Tbsp	curry powder
½ tsp	kosher salt
½ tsp	ground pepper
1 cup	low-sodium chicken broth
	Juice of ½ lemon

1 Boil unpeeled yams until just tender. Drain and cool.

2 Peel and chop the yams and set aside.

3 Sauté the chopped onion in the olive oil. Add the spices and chicken broth, and bring to a boil.

4 Add the cooked yams. Cover and simmer over low heat until the yams are tender (about 5 minutes). Sprinkle with the lemon juice before serving.

CHEF'S NOTES: Substitute vegetable broth in this recipe to make it vegetarian friendly. Yams and sweet potatoes are a good source of manganese. There is some evidence that having too little manganese in a person's system may impact blood glucose.

Exchanges/Food Choices
1 1/2 Starch   1/2 Fat

Basic Nutritional Values

Calories	120
Calories from Fat	30
Total Fat	3.5 g
Saturated Fat	0.6 g
Trans Fat	0.0 g
Cholesterol	0 mg
Sodium	160 mg
Potassium	300 mg
Total Carbohydrate	20 g
Dietary Fiber	3 g
Sugars	7 g
Protein	2 g
Phosphorus	45 mg

I have heard that when you went to the movies back in the day, there would be a cartoon, then news, a B movie, and then the feature film. And back in the day people just referred to diabetes as "sugar" and tried to cut down on sweets.

Well, times have changed. Now you get to see a dozen coming attractions and one movie and the prices are rising at a steady pace. The rates of obesity and diabetes are also rising at an astronomical rate. We know things must change. We know we must change them.

Main dishes are not, as I used to believe, the feature attraction of our daily food intake. They are part of the whole picture. We need to step back and plan ahead to make sure we have the balance of nutrients our bodies require throughout the day.

The foods in this section will take you on a journey from Jamaica to Cuba to China . . . all around the globe. The cuisine of my mother's homeland of Jamaica has been influenced over the years by the foods of many lands. In the 1500s the Spanish took the land from the Arawak peoples. In the years that followed, British, Chinese, Portuguese, French, Dutch, and East Indian ingredients and styles of cooking all helped to form what we recognize today as Jamaican food. You will see those influences in this chapter.

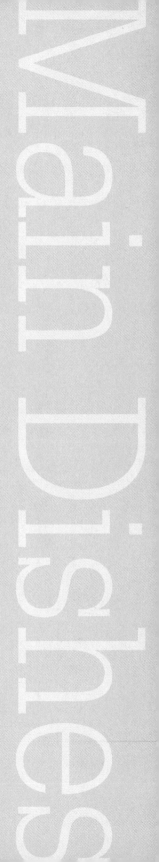

Turkey Curry Made with Yogurt

Crunchy Lime Pepper Baked Catfish with Brown Rice

Spicy Fish and Collard Greens

Country Captain

Citrus-Baked Pork Chops

Egg Foo Yung

Chickpea Casserole

Broiled Tilapia with Plum Sauce

Easy Eggplant Bake

Chicken Brown-Rice Salad

Easiest Chicken Salad Ever

Curried Chicken Salad with Baby Spinach

Spinach-Wrapped Chicken

Curry Dipping Sauce

Cold Spiced Salmon

Baked Fish with Citrus and Herbs

Chicken Lover Balsamic Chicken

Cod Provençale

Fiesta Fish Tacos

Mexican Turkey Burgers

Moroccan Lamb Stew with Apricots

Open-Faced Greek Burgers

Brown Rice "Porcupine" Meatballs

Chicken and Chickpeas with Lemon and Garlic

Thai Chicken Kabobs with Peanut Butter Dipping Sauce

Peanut Butter Dipping Sauce

Cuban Roasted Pork Loin

Peppers Stuffed with Rice and Greens

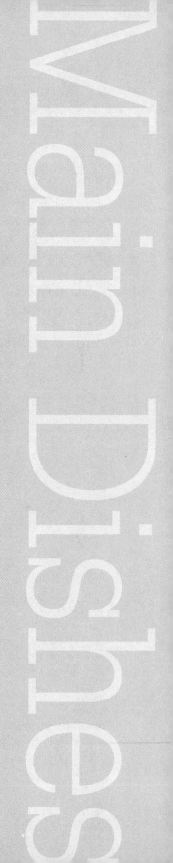

Turkey Curry Made with Yogurt

SERVES 6   **SERVING SIZE** 1/6th recipe

2	medium onions, diced
1 Tbsp	olive oil
1	large clove garlic, minced
2 Tbsp	curry powder (more or less to taste)
2 tsp	powdered ginger
2 tsp	cinnamon
1 tsp	black pepper
1 tsp	cayenne pepper
1 tsp	cumin
1	(2-lb) package turkey breast cutlets, cut into bite-size pieces
1	(16-oz) container plain, nonfat yogurt

1. Using a large skillet over medium heat, sauté the diced onion in the olive oil until transparent.

2. Add the garlic, curry powder, and spices. Stir in the spices so that the pan of onions is seasoned and golden.

3. Push the seasoned onions to the side of the pan and add the pieces of turkey.

4. When the turkey pieces are cooked through, mix them into the spiced onions and turn off the heat.

5. Let sit 5 minutes to cool slightly, then spoon in the yogurt, mixing to make a sauce. Note: if the meat/onion mixture is too hot, the yogurt will curdle.

OPTIONAL GARNISHES:
- Toasted unsweetened coconut
- Chopped unsalted peanuts
- Raisins

Exchanges/Food Choices
1/2 Fat-Free Milk   1 Vegetable   4 Lean Meat

Basic Nutritional Values

Calories	250
Calories from Fat	35
Total Fat	4.0 g
Saturated Fat	0.8 g
Trans Fat	0.0 g
Cholesterol	100 mg
Sodium	115 mg
Potassium	650 mg
Total Carbohydrate	13 g
Dietary Fiber	2 g
Sugars	7 g
Protein	41 g
Phosphorus	415 mg

CHEF'S NOTES: Boneless, skinless chicken breasts can be substituted for the turkey if you prefer. I just go to my freezer, pull out one of my bags of precooked, cubed chicken breast and I am ready to go. To keep the mixture from curdling when the yogurt is added, be sure to follow the direction to cool the curry a bit. Then empty the yogurt into a bowl and stir in a few spoonfuls of the curry. Add this all back into the pot and it will be smooth and ready to eat.

Crunchy Lime Pepper Baked Catfish with Brown Rice

SERVES 4

Nonstick cooking spray
1 lb catfish fillets
2 limes
¼ cup dried bread crumbs
½ tsp black pepper
½ tsp salt (optional)
2 Tbsp olive oil
2 cups cooked brown rice

1. Coat bottom of glass baking dish with nonstick cooking spray.

2. Pat fish fillets with paper towel and place in baking dish.

3. Squeeze juice of 2 limes over fish. Mix bread crumbs, black pepper, and salt (if desired). Pat onto fish. Drizzle with olive oil.

4. Bake at 325°F until fish flakes easily (6–10 minutes).

5. Divide into 4 portions. Serve each portion over 1/2 cup of brown rice.

CHEF'S NOTES: I like to have a big dish of assorted steamed vegetables to round out this meal. They say fish is "brain food." I think fish is a smart choice, especially for people with diabetes.

Exchanges/Food Choices
2 Starch   3 Lean Meat   1 1/2 Fat

Basic Nutritional Values

Calories	345
Calories from Fat	135
Total Fat	15.0 g
Saturated Fat	2.8 g
Trans Fat	0.1 g
Cholesterol	65 mg
Sodium	180 mg
Potassium	445 mg
Total Carbohydrate	29 g
Dietary Fiber	2 g
Sugars	1 g
Protein	22 g
Phosphorus	345 mg

Spicy Fish and Collard Greens

SERVES 4   **SERVING SIZE** 1/4th recipe

1	large bunch collard greens (about 1½ lb)
1 cup plus 3 Tbsp	water, divided use
3 Tbsp	olive oil
1 large	green pepper, diced
1 large	onion, diced
1 lb	fish fillets, cut into strips (use any available whitefish)
½ tsp	kosher salt
½ tsp	ground black pepper
¼ tsp	cayenne pepper
Dash	red pepper flakes

1. Clean and trim collard greens, then chop coarsely.

2. Bring 1 cup water to boil. Add collard greens and continue boiling for 15–20 minutes until the greens are soft. Drain and set aside.

3. Mix the olive oil and the remaining 3 Tbsp of water in a heavy saucepan. Add the collard greens, chopped pepper, and chopped onion. Cook for 5–7 minutes, stirring occasionally, until the onions are transparent but still a bit crisp.

4. Add the strips of fish. Sprinkle with the salt, pepper, and cayenne. Cover and simmer until the fish is flakey, about 7 minutes.

5. Sprinkle with red pepper flakes before serving.

Exchanges/Food Choices
3 Vegetable   3 Lean Meat   1 Fat

Basic Nutritional Values

Calories	255
Calories from Fat	110
Total Fat	12.0 g
Saturated Fat	1.7 g
Trans Fat	0.0 g
Cholesterol	65 mg
Sodium	340 mg
Potassium	665 mg
Total Carbohydrate	14 g
Dietary Fiber	5 g
Sugars	4 g
Protein	25 g
Phosphorus	275 mg

CHEF'S NOTES: You can use any mild-flavored, firm white fish in this recipe. Haddock or monkfish are good choices but can be pricey. Watch for sales but purchase only what you are going to use right away. Don't be surprised at how much your large bunch of greens will cook down. I like to combine different types, such as kale and turnip greens, to vary the flavor.

Country Captain

SERVES 6

SERVING SIZE 1/6th recipe

1	(32-oz) package boneless, skinless chicken breasts
¼ cup	canola oil
1	(28-oz) can chopped tomatoes, undrained
2	medium onions, chopped
2	medium green peppers, chopped
2	cloves garlic, minced
2	bay leaves, crushed
½ tsp	ground pepper
½ tsp	kosher salt
½ tsp	powdered thyme
2 tsp	curry powder

1 Preheat oven to 325°F.

2 Sauté the chicken breasts in the canola oil until just barely cooked. Set cooked chicken aside.

3 Add all the remaining ingredients to the saucepan used to cook the chicken. Mix well and simmer for 10 minutes.

4 Put chicken breasts in a baking pan and cover with the tomato mixture.

5 Cover pan and bake until the chicken is very tender, about 55 minutes.

6 Serve with brown rice or over whole-wheat pasta. This dish is traditionally garnished with currants and peanuts or almonds.

Exchanges/Food Choices
2 Vegetable   4 Lean Meat   1 1/2 Fat

Basic Nutritional Values

Calories	300
Calories from Fat	115
Total Fat	13.0 g
Saturated Fat	1.8 g
Trans Fat	0.0 g
Cholesterol	90 mg
Sodium	350 mg
Potassium	590 mg
Total Carbohydrate	11 g
Dietary Fiber	3 g
Sugars	5 g
Protein	34 g
Phosphorus	280 mg

CHEF'S NOTES: When tomatoes are plentiful and economical it is a good time to buy them by the bushel and can them for use all year round. If you purchase canned tomatoes at your grocery store, please check the label and watch for added sugar.

Citrus-Baked Pork Chops

6	lean, center-cut pork chops (36 oz total)
1 tsp	salt-free lemon pepper
2 Tbsp	olive oil
1	lemon, cut into six round slices
½ cup	ketchup (preferably no-sugar)
½ cup	water
1 tsp	hot pepper sauce
Dash	salt

1. Preheat oven to 375°F.

2. Sprinkle meat with the lemon pepper.

3. Heat the oil in a heavy frying pan and brown the chops on both sides.

4. Drain fat and arrange in a baking dish. Place a slice of lemon on each chop.

5. Combine ketchup, water, and pepper sauce, pour over chops.

6. Bake until tender but no longer pink, about 50 minutes.

CHEF'S NOTES: Today's pork is leaner than ever before. Leaner can sometimes mean dryer, but cooking it in this lemony tomato sauce will keep it moist and flavorful. If 1 tsp of pepper sauce is enough for you, that is fine. If not, join me and add a couple more.

Exchanges/Food Choices
1/2 Carbohydrate   3 Lean Meat   1 Fat

Basic Nutritional Values

Calories	220
Calories from Fat	100
Total Fat	11.0 g
Saturated Fat	3.1 g
Trans Fat	0.0 g
Cholesterol	70 mg
Sodium	305 mg
Potassium	390 mg
Total Carbohydrate	5 g
Dietary Fiber	0 g
Sugars	5 g
Protein	25 g
Phosphorus	160 mg

Egg Foo Yung

SERVES 8

¾	cup low-sodium chicken broth
2 Tbsp	reduced-sodium soy sauce
¾ tsp	ground ginger
½ tsp	hot pepper sauce
½ tsp	garlic powder
1 Tbsp	cornstarch
½ tsp	dark sesame oil
½ cup	water
3	large eggs
6	egg whites
½ cup	cubed cooked pork loin (or chicken)
3	green onions, thinly sliced
½ lb	bean sprouts, chopped
1	medium carrot, shredded
¼ lb	brown mushrooms, chopped
4 Tbsp	canola oil, divided use

1. In a large saucepan, combine chicken broth, soy sauce, ginger, hot pepper, garlic powder, cornstarch, sesame oil, and water. Cook over medium heat, stirring constantly, until the sauce has thickened. Cover and keep sauce warm.

2. Beat eggs and egg whites until frothy. Add meat, onions, bean sprouts, and carrot to the egg mixture.

3. In a separate saucepan, sauté the mushrooms in 2 Tbsp of oil. Drain and add mushrooms to the egg mixture.

4. Heat remaining oil in the frying pan. When it is hot, add the egg mixture as if making pancakes, approximately 1/4 cup at a time.

5. Cook patties until golden brown, turning once.

6. Remove patties from heat and pour the warm sauce over them before serving.

Exchanges/Food Choices
1 Vegetable   1 Lean Meat   1 1/2 Fat

Basic Nutritional Values

Calories	130
Calories from Fat	70
Total Fat	8.0 g
Saturated Fat	1.4 g
Trans Fat	0.0 g
Cholesterol	75 mg
Sodium	230 mg
Potassium	260 mg
Total Carbohydrate	5 g
Dietary Fiber	1 g
Sugars	2 g
Protein	9 g
Phosphorus	100 mg

CHEF'S NOTES: From take-out to take a bow! Make this and congratulate yourself for saving money and creating a filling, delicious, healthy meal. It is a great way to use up leftovers. A bottle of dark sesame oil is a wonderful investment. You will be amazed by how much flavor just a little bit of this oil will add.

Chickpea Casserole

2	large onions, minced
2 Tbsp	olive oil
3	cloves garlic, minced
2 tsp	cumin
2 tsp	curry powder
3	baby eggplants, unpeeled and sliced
1 cup	low-sodium vegetable broth or chicken broth
4 cups	cooked chickpeas
½ tsp	salt

1 Sauté onions in olive oil until softened, then add the garlic, cumin, curry powder, and eggplant. Cook for 5 minutes over medium heat.

2 Add broth, chickpeas, and salt. Simmer for 15 minutes.

CHEF'S NOTES: I like to cook this the day before I plan to eat it and let it sit in the refrigerator overnight. That way the chickpeas take on all the flavors of the other ingredients.

Exchanges/Food Choices
2 Starch   3 Vegetable   1 Fat

Basic Nutritional Values

Calories	275
Calories from Fat	70
Total Fat	8.0 g
Saturated Fat	1.0 g
Trans Fat	0.0 g
Cholesterol	0 mg
Sodium	230 mg
Potassium	540 mg
Total Carbohydrate	43 g
Dietary Fiber	11 g
Sugars	10 g
Protein	11 g
Phosphorus	235 mg

Broiled Tilapia with Plum Sauce

SERVES 4   **SERVING SIZE** 1/4th recipe

1 lb	tilapia fillets
2 Tbsp	olive oil
1 tsp	salt-free lemon pepper seasoning
¾ lb	plums
1 cup	water
1 tsp	rice wine vinegar
2	cloves garlic, minced

1 Place tilapia fillets on a broiler pan covered with nonstick aluminum foil.

2 Drizzle with olive oil and sprinkle with lemon pepper seasoning.

3 Broil until fish flakes easily. Depending on thickness of fish, this could take 5–8 minutes.

4 Slice, pit, and chop plums. Put into saucepan with water, vinegar, and garlic. Simmer for 10 minutes.

5 Spoon 2 Tbsp of sauce over each fillet.

CHEF'S NOTES: Tilapia is a mild white fish that is an excellent canvas for the sweet and spicy plum sauce. This sauce also goes well with chicken or pork.

Exchanges/Food Choices
1/2 Fruit   3 Lean Meat   1 Fat

Basic Nutritional Values

Calories	210
Calories from Fat	80
Total Fat	9.0 g
Saturated Fat	1.8 g
Trans Fat	0.0 g
Cholesterol	50 mg
Sodium	50 mg
Potassium	460 mg
Total Carbohydrate	10 g
Dietary Fiber	1 g
Sugars	8 g
Protein	23 g
Phosphorus	190 mg

Easy Eggplant Bake

2	medium eggplant (about 1¼ lb each), peeled and cut into slices
2	medium onions, diced
1	clove garlic, minced
2 Tbsp	plus 1 tsp olive oil, divided use
¼ tsp	ground pepper
¼ tsp	fennel seed
1 Tbsp	chopped fresh dill (or 1 tsp dried dill)
½ tsp	fresh mint
½ cup	water or low-sodium vegetable broth
6	firm Roma tomatoes, sliced

1. Preheat oven to 400°F.

2. Lightly sprinkle kosher salt on the eggplant slices. After they "sweat," rinse, drain, pat dry, and layer them in a glass baking dish.

3. Sauté the onions and garlic in 2 Tbsp of olive oil. Add the spices and herbs and the water. Bring to a boil.

4. Using a colander, drain the liquid and add it to the eggplant slices.

5. Bake at 400°F for 10 minutes. Reduce oven heat to 350°F.

6. Spoon the spiced onion mixture left in the colander over the eggplant slices. Add the tomato slices. Drizzle the remaining 1 tsp olive oil on top and bake for another hour.

Exchanges/Food Choices
2 Vegetable   1/2 Fat

Basic Nutritional Values

Calories	75
Calories from Fat	30
Total Fat	3.5 g
Saturated Fat	0.5 g
Trans Fat	0.0 g
Cholesterol	0 mg
Sodium	100 mg
Potassium	240 mg
Total Carbohydrate	12 g
Dietary Fiber	3 g
Sugars	5 g
Protein	1 g
Phosphorus	30 mg

CHEF'S NOTES: Eggplant is low in calories but high in fiber. It does have a high salt content, which makes it important to rinse it off after using salt to pull out excess moisture.

Chicken Brown-Rice Salad

SERVES 6   **SERVING SIZE** 1 chicken breast half and 1 cup rice salad

2/3 cup   bottled fat-free Italian salad dressing, divided use

6   small skinless, boneless chicken breast halves (about 1½ lb total)

1 cup   loosely packed frozen French-cut green beans

3 cups   cooked brown rice, chilled

1   (14-oz) can artichoke hearts, drained and quartered

2 cups   coleslaw mix (shredded cabbage with carrot)

6   lettuce leaves

1. Place 3 Tbsp of the Italian salad dressing in a small bowl. Set aside remaining Italian salad dressing.

2. Place chicken on the rack of an uncovered grill directly over medium coals. Grill for 12–15 minutes or until chicken is tender and no longer pink (170°F), turning once and brushing with the 3 Tbsp of dressing during the last 2 minutes.

3. Rinse green beans with cool water for 30 seconds; drain well. In a large bowl toss together beans, chilled rice, artichoke hearts, and coleslaw mix. Pour the reserved salad dressing over rice mixture; toss to gently coat.

4. Remove chicken from grill and slice. Arrange lettuce leaves on 6 dinner plates. Top with the rice mixture and chicken slices.

Exchanges/Food Choices
1 1/2 Starch   2 Vegetable   3 Lean Meat

Basic Nutritional Values

Calories	290
Calories from Fat	35
Total Fat	4.0 g
Saturated Fat	1.1 g
Trans Fat	0.0 g
Cholesterol	65 mg
Sodium	480 mg
Potassium	475 mg
Total Carbohydrate	32 g
Dietary Fiber	5 g
Sugars	3 g
Protein	29 g
Phosphorus	330 mg

CHEF'S NOTES: Simple, quick, and healthy—a recipe triple play! Artichoke hearts, green beans, and shredded cabbage and carrots help make this whole-grain chicken salad a home run for everyone in your home. Using French-cut green beans gives more surface to lightly coat with the tangy dressing. Great fiber in the cabbage and carrots helps the body in so many ways. And artichokes are known to reduce cholesterol, improve digestion, and make your gallbladder function better.

Easiest Chicken Salad Ever

SERVES 4

½ **cup** plain, nonfat Greek-style yogurt
1 **Tbsp** Dijon mustard
½ **tsp** ground black pepper
2 **cups** chopped cooked chicken
½ **cup** sliced almonds

1. Combine the yogurt, mustard, and pepper.

2. Mix in the chicken and sliced almonds.

3. Chill before serving on a bed of salad greens.

CHEF'S NOTES: Thaw a package of frozen, precooked chicken breast cubes and you can have this made in minutes. Remember, 1/4 of your plate should contain meat or a meat substitute, 1/4 should be complex carbs, and 1/2 of your plate should contain vegetables. With all the choices available in your farmers market, finding vegetables to complement this chicken salad won't be difficult.

Exchanges/Food Choices
4 Lean Meat   1/2 Fat

Basic Nutritional Values

Calories	200	
Calories from Fat	70	
Total Fat	8.0	g
Saturated Fat	1.1	g
Trans Fat	0.0	g
Cholesterol	60	mg
Sodium	155	mg
Potassium	295	mg
Total Carbohydrate	4	g
Dietary Fiber	1	g
Sugars	2	g
Protein	27	g
Phosphorus	250	mg

Curried Chicken Salad with Baby Spinach

SERVES 4

SERVING SIZE 1/4th recipe

1 Tbsp	curry powder
1 cup	plain, nonfat yogurt
½ cup	mandarin oranges packed in water, drained
2 cups	cubed cooked chicken breast
1	bunch (about 10 oz) baby spinach, raw
¼ cup	slivered almonds

1 Mix curry powder into yogurt.

2 Gently fold in oranges and chicken.

3 Place chicken salad on baby spinach leaves and top with slivered almonds.

CHEF'S NOTES: Sweet and spicy and so quick to put together. Watch for boneless, skinless chicken breasts to go on sale. Bake or poach. Cut into cubes and freeze in 2-cup portions. You can buy a bag of prewashed baby spinach and use half for this recipe and half for another, such as Chicken and Chickpeas with Lemon and Garlic (page 119).

Exchanges/Food Choices
1 Carbohydrate   3 Lean Meat

Basic Nutritional Values

Calories	215
Calories from Fat	65
Total Fat	7.0 g
Saturated Fat	1.1 g
Trans Fat	0.0 g
Cholesterol	60 mg
Sodium	135 mg
Potassium	720 mg
Total Carbohydrate	11 g
Dietary Fiber	3 g
Sugars	7 g
Protein	28 g
Phosphorus	325 mg

Spinach-Wrapped Chicken

SERVES 8

1 lb	spinach (stems removed)
2	quarts boiling water
1	(10.75-oz) can low-sodium chicken broth
¼ cup	reduced-sodium soy sauce
1	clove garlic, minced
1 Tbsp	Worcestershire sauce
1	(32-oz) package boneless, skinless chicken breasts
1 cup	Curry Dipping Sauce (page 109)

1. Wash spinach and place in metal colander and pour boiling water over the spinach leaves. Drain and set aside to cool.

2. Combine chicken broth, soy sauce, garlic, and Worcestershire sauce. Bring to a boil in a large frying pan.

3. Cut chicken breasts into large cubes (about 2 inches). Add to liquid, reduce heat, and simmer until chicken is cooked through. Drain chicken and set aside to cool.

4. Wrap each cube in a spinach leaf, securing with a toothpick and refrigerate for a day.

5. Serve with Curry Dipping Sauce.

Exchanges/Food Choices
1/2 Carbohydrate   3 Lean Meat

Basic Nutritional Values

Calories	170
Calories from Fat	25
Total Fat	3.0 g
Saturated Fat	1.1 g
Trans Fat	0.0 g
Cholesterol	65 mg
Sodium	320 mg
Potassium	450 mg
Total Carbohydrate	7 g
Dietary Fiber	1 g
Sugars	3 g
Protein	27 g
Phosphorus	180 mg

Curry Dipping Sauce

¼ **cup**   plain, nonfat Greek-style yogurt
¼ **cup**   light sour cream
 2 tsp   curry powder
3 Tbsp   mango chutney (Major Grey's), chopped
 1 tsp   grated orange peel
 Dash   dried red pepper flakes

1 Combine all ingredients and mix well.

2 Cover and chill for at least 2 hours.

CHEF'S NOTES: Although my recipe calls for chutney, I often substitute 3 Tbsp of well-drained, no-sugar-added, crushed pineapple. Chutney adds an interesting flavor but is also more expensive than the pineapple. Just use a small amount of the dipping sauce per serving.

Exchanges/Food Choices
1/2 Carbohydrate

Basic Nutritional Values

Calories	25
Calories from Fat	0
Total Fat	0.0 g
Saturated Fat	0.3 g
Trans Fat	0.0 g
Cholesterol	0 mg
Sodium	50 mg
Potassium	30 mg
Total Carbohydrate	4 g
Dietary Fiber	0 g
Sugars	3 g
Protein	1 g
Phosphorus	15 mg

Cold Spiced Salmon

½ cup	white wine vinegar
¼ cup	fresh lemon juice
¼ cup	olive oil
1	small onion, sliced very thin
2	cloves garlic, crushed
3	dried bay leaves, crushed
1 tsp	whole mustard seeds
½ tsp	kosher salt
1 tsp	whole black peppercorns
2 lb	boned and skinned salmon, lightly poached and cut into cubes

1. Combine all ingredients except the salmon in a saucepan and bring to a boil.

2. Place salmon cubes in a glass bowl and then pour the hot marinade over the fish, making sure all the cubes are covered.

3. Cover and refrigerate for 24 hours.

4. Drain and serve over lettuce as a salad or with toothpicks as an appetizer.

CHEF'S NOTES: Leftovers are perfect used in some of the breakfast recipes that call for salmon.

Exchanges/Food Choices
3 Lean Meat   1 1/2 Fat

Basic Nutritional Values

Calories	200
Calories from Fat	90
Total Fat	10.0 g
Saturated Fat	1.9 g
Trans Fat	0.0 g
Cholesterol	50 mg
Sodium	110 mg
Potassium	425 mg
Total Carbohydrate	1 g
Dietary Fiber	0 g
Sugars	0 g
Protein	24 g
Phosphorus	270 mg

Baked Fish with Citrus and Herbs

SERVES 6

Nonstick cooking spray
1½ lb   mild white fish (halibut, cod, or tilapia)
2 Tbsp   olive oil
2 Tbsp   fresh lemon juice
2   cloves garlic, minced
1 Tbsp   fines herbes (can substitute 1 Tbsp dried parsley)
½ tsp   thyme
½ tsp   ground white pepper
¼ cup   grated reduced-fat Parmesan cheese for topping
Thinly sliced lemon (for garnish)

1   Preheat oven to 425°F.

2   Treat a 13 × 9-inch glass baking dish with nonstick cooking spray.

3   Arrange the fish fillets in a single layer in the baking dish.

4   Mix the olive oil, lemon juice, garlic, fines herbes, thyme, and pepper. Pour evenly over the fish. Sprinkle lightly with Parmesan cheese.

5   Bake until fish is done, about 20 minutes. (Be careful not to overcook.)

6   Garnish with thinly sliced rounds of lemon.

CHEF'S NOTES: Island cuisine calls for quite a bit of fish. Use whatever white fish is on sale. Fish can be a real bargain. There is little shrinkage or waste. And it is so good for you.

Exchanges/Food Choices
4 Lean Meat

Basic Nutritional Values

Calories	185
Calories from Fat	70
Total Fat	8.0 g
Saturated Fat	1.5 g
Trans Fat	0.0 g
Cholesterol	40 mg
Sodium	145 mg
Potassium	535 mg
Total Carbohydrate	3 g
Dietary Fiber	0 g
Sugars	0 g
Protein	25 g
Phosphorus	290 mg

Chicken Lover Balsamic Chicken

4	small skinless, boneless chicken breast halves (about 1 lb total)
1 Tbsp	paprika
1 Tbsp	olive oil
½ tsp	snipped fresh rosemary
2	cloves garlic, minced
¼ tsp	ground black pepper
	Nonstick cooking spray
¼ cup	dry red wine or water
3 Tbsp	balsamic vinegar
	Fresh rosemary sprigs (optional, for garnish)

1. If desired, place each chicken breast half between 2 pieces of plastic wrap and pound with the flat side of a meat mallet to a rectangle 1/4- to 1/2-inch thick.

2. In a small bowl, combine paprika, oil, rosemary, garlic, and pepper; mix well until it becomes a paste. Rub both sides of each chicken breast half with paste mixture.

3. Coat a 13 × 9 × 2-inch baking pan with nonstick cooking spray. Place coated chicken in prepared pan; cover and refrigerate for 2–6 hours.

4. Preheat oven to 450°F.

5. Drizzle chicken with wine. Bake for 10–12 minutes or until an instant-read meat thermometer inserted in the thickest portion of the chicken registers 170°F and the juices run clear, turning once halfway through baking. (If chicken has been pounded, bake about 6 minutes or until chicken is no longer pink and juices run clear, turning once halfway through baking.)

6. Remove from oven. Immediately drizzle vinegar onto chicken in the baking pan.

7. Transfer chicken to serving plates. Stir the liquid in the baking pan and drizzle over chicken. If desired, garnish with fresh rosemary.

CHEF'S NOTES: Many people who have changed their diet will stick to chicken and fish and some beef. This is a tasty dish for those chicken lovers who want to put a simple twist on a chicken recipe. A rub seasoned with paprika, rosemary, and garlic gives this low-calorie chicken recipe lively flavor while a balsamic vinegar drizzle adds subtle sweetness.

Exchanges/Food Choices
4 Lean Meat

Basic Nutritional Values

Calories	180
Calories from Fat	55
Total Fat	6.0 g
Saturated Fat	1.3 g
Trans Fat	0.0 g
Cholesterol	65 mg
Sodium	60 mg
Potassium	265 mg
Total Carbohydrate	3 g
Dietary Fiber	1 g
Sugars	2 g
Protein	24 g
Phosphorus	185 mg

Cod Provençale

Nonstick cooking spray
2½ Tbsp olive oil
1 large onion, diced
3 cloves garlic, minced
1 large bell pepper, diced
1 (2-oz) can anchovies packed in oil, chopped and drained but not rinsed
½ cup pitted black olives
⅛ tsp fennel seed
¼ tsp ground black pepper
8 boneless cod steaks (3 lb total)
4 tomato slices
2 Tbsp tomato paste, diluted with water to make ½ cup
1 cup red wine

1 Preheat oven to 375°F.

2 Prep a baking dish with nonstick cooking spray.

3 Heat the olive oil in a heavy skillet and add onions, garlic, and bell pepper, cooking until the onion is soft. Add the anchovies, olives, fennel seed, and black pepper. Stir to combine.

4 Place 4 pieces of the cod in a single layer in the baking dish. Spread evenly with the anchovy/olive mixture.

5 Top each piece with another piece, making a cod "sandwich." Top each with a slice of tomato.

6 Combine the diluted tomato paste with the red wine and pour over the fish.

7 Bake for 20 minutes until the fish is flaky, basting every 5 minutes or so.

Exchanges/Food Choices
1 Vegetable   4 Lean Meat

Basic Nutritional Values

Calories	230
Calories from Fat	65
Total Fat	7.0 g
Saturated Fat	1.1 g
Trans Fat	0.0 g
Cholesterol	80 mg
Sodium	425 mg
Potassium	520 mg
Total Carbohydrate	6 g
Dietary Fiber	2 g
Sugars	3 g
Protein	33 g
Phosphorus	220 mg

CHEF'S NOTES: I rarely use anchovies but they do add an interesting flavor to this cod dish. If you decide to omit them, use one small roasted red pepper chopped fine.

Fiesta Fish Tacos

	Juice of ½ lime
2	cloves garlic, minced
1 Tbsp	olive oil
1 lb	tilapia fillets
½ cup	chopped green bell pepper
½ cup	chopped red bell pepper
1 Tbsp	minced cilantro
1 cup	cherry or grape tomatoes
4	(6-inch) whole-wheat tortillas
2 cups	shredded lettuce
1 cup	cubed mango
	Black pepper, to taste

1. Mix lime juice, garlic, and olive oil in a glass bowl.

2. Add tilapia and marinate in refrigerator for 1 hour.

3. Place tilapia in a glass baking dish surrounded by green and red bell pepper, minced cilantro, and tomatoes.

4. Bake at 350°F for 10 minutes or until fish flakes easily.

5. Divide fish and veggies into 4 servings and place on each of the warmed tortillas.

6. Top with lettuce, cubed mango, and a sprinkling of black pepper.

CHEF'S NOTES: These tacos are filling and satisfying. I enjoy the combination of the mild fish, the tangy marinade, and the sweetness of the tomatoes and mango.

Exchanges/Food Choices

1 Starch   1/2 Fruit   1 Vegetable   3 Lean Meat

Basic Nutritional Values

Calories	260
Calories from Fat	55
Total Fat	6.0 g
Saturated Fat	1.4 g
Trans Fat	0.0 g
Cholesterol	50 mg
Sodium	190 mg
Potassium	675 mg
Total Carbohydrate	27 g
Dietary Fiber	4 g
Sugars	9 g
Protein	26 g
Phosphorus	260 mg

Mexican Turkey Burgers

SERVES 4

1 lb	(93%) lean ground turkey
2	cloves garlic, minced
1	medium purple onion, finely diced
½	medium green pepper, finely diced
½ tsp	ground black pepper
1 tsp	cumin
½ Tbsp	chili pepper
1 Tbsp	olive oil

1. Combine all ingredients except the olive oil, being careful not to overmix.

2. Separate the meat mixture into 4 balls and flatten into patties.

3. Heat olive oil in skillet and sauté burgers until done.

4. Serve without buns.

CHEF'S NOTES: Cumin adds a smoky flavor to the ground turkey. The turkey has very little fat. The onion and green pepper add moisture, which will help keep these burgers from being too dry.

Exchanges/Food Choices
1 Vegetable   3 Lean Meat   1 1/2 Fat

Basic Nutritional Values

Calories	230
Calories from Fat	115
Total Fat	13.0 g
Saturated Fat	3.0 g
Trans Fat	0.1 g
Cholesterol	85 mg
Sodium	85 mg
Potassium	370 mg
Total Carbohydrate	6 g
Dietary Fiber	1 g
Sugars	2 g
Protein	23 g
Phosphorus	235 mg

Moroccan Lamb Stew with Apricots

SERVES 6

1 lb	boneless leg of lamb
½ tsp	kosher salt
	Nonstick cooking spray
2	medium onions, diced
1½ tsp	ground cumin
½ tsp	ground chili pepper
¾ tsp	cinnamon
6	cloves garlic, minced
1 Tbsp	blue agave syrup
1 Tbsp	tomato paste
½ cup	dried apricots, cut in quarters
1	(14-oz) can low-sodium beef broth

1. Trim the fat from the lamb and cut it into small cubes. Sprinkle with the salt.

2. Prepare a Dutch oven with nonstick cooking spray and heat over medium heat.

3. Brown the cubes of lamb on all sides in the Dutch oven. Remove the lamb and set aside.

4. Brown the onion in the lamb drippings. Add the cumin, pepper, cinnamon, and garlic.

5. Stir the onions and spices for a minute, then add the agave syrup and tomato paste. Add the sautéed lamb, the apricots, and the broth.

6. Bring to a boil, then reduce heat and simmer, covered, until the lamb is tender (about an hour). Stir occasionally.

7. Serve with couscous or triangles of pita bread.

Exchanges/Food Choices
1 Carbohydrate   2 Lean Meat   1/2 Fat

Basic Nutritional Values

Calories	195
Calories from Fat	55
Total Fat	6.0 g
Saturated Fat	2.0 g
Trans Fat	0.0 g
Cholesterol	55 mg
Sodium	265 mg
Potassium	515 mg
Total Carbohydrate	17 g
Dietary Fiber	2 g
Sugars	12 g
Protein	19 g
Phosphorus	165 mg

CHEF'S NOTES: I love Moroccan cooking. Lamb is used often and is delicious in this dish and many others. Lamb can be expensive, though. Watch for sales but feel free to substitute a pound of cubed chicken breast if you like. You will need to add 1 Tbsp of olive oil to replace the fat that would have been provided by the lamb.

Open-Faced Greek Burgers

SERVES 4

1 pound	lean ground beef (95% or higher)
2 tsp	minced garlic
1 tsp	garlic powder
1 tsp	onion powder
2 tsp	cumin
1 tsp	salt-free lemon pepper seasoning
½ tsp	sea salt

1 Mix beef and seasonings. Form into 4 patties.

2 Preheat broiler in oven.

3 Place patties on broiler pan and cook for 4 minutes per side.

4 Remove from oven and place on paper towels to drain any excess fat.

5 Serve on 1/2 oval-shaped, whole-wheat flat bread (optional). Top with 1 Tbsp yogurt sauce (optional).

CHEF'S NOTES: Yes, people with diabetes can have burgers when they are filled with flavor not fat. These burgers are so tasty even your friends and family members without diabetes will be begging for the recipe.

Exchanges/Food Choices
1/2 Carbohydrate   4 Lean Meat

Basic Nutritional Values

Calories	210
Calories from Fat	65
Total Fat	7.0 g
Saturated Fat	3.4 g
Trans Fat	0.2 g
Cholesterol	70 mg
Sodium	390 mg
Potassium	535 mg
Total Carbohydrate	7 g
Dietary Fiber	1 g
Sugars	4 g
Protein	29 g
Phosphorus	300 mg

YOGURT SAUCE

1 cup	plain, low-fat Greek-style yogurt
1 cup	diced cucumber
¼ cup	diced purple onion
2 Tbsp	lemon juice

1 Mix yogurt, cucumber, onion, and lemon juice and let sit while preparing the burgers.

Brown Rice "Porcupine" Meatballs

SERVES 4

SERVING SIZE 2 meatballs

1 lb	lean ground beef (at least 95%)
1 cup	cooked brown rice, chilled
1 cup	chopped onion
1 tsp	smoked paprika
1 tsp	black pepper
1 tsp	garlic powder
1	egg, beaten
16 oz	low-sodium vegetable juice

1 Preheat oven to 350°F.

2 Mix beef, rice, onion, seasonings, and beaten egg.

3 Form into 8 meatballs.

4 Place meatballs in baking dish, add the vegetable juice, and bake for 30 minutes.

5 Serve with a green salad dressed with a little olive oil and lemon juice, if desired.

CHEF'S NOTES: The old-fashioned recipe for these meatballs used white rice and canned tomato soup. My tweaks make it healthier, more nutritious, and even tastier.

Exchanges/Food Choices
1 Starch   1 Vegetable   3 Lean Meat   1/2 Fat

Basic Nutritional Values

Calories	265
Calories from Fat	70
Total Fat	8.0 g
Saturated Fat	3.2 g
Trans Fat	0.2 g
Cholesterol	115 mg
Sodium	160 mg
Potassium	710 mg
Total Carbohydrate	21 g
Dietary Fiber	3 g
Sugars	6 g
Protein	27 g
Phosphorus	305 mg

Chicken and Chickpeas with Lemon and Garlic

SERVES 4

½ **cup**	chopped purple onion
2	cloves garlic, chopped
1 **Tbsp**	olive oil
1 **cup**	canned chickpeas, drained and rinsed
2 **cups**	cubed cooked chicken breast
½	(16-oz) bag baby spinach
	Juice of ½ lemon
⅓ **cup**	reduced-fat feta crumbles

1 Sauté onion and garlic in olive oil on medium heat until onion softens.

2 Add chickpeas and chicken and cook over low heat for 5 minutes.

3 Add half bag of baby spinach (left over from Curried Chicken Salad recipe, page 107). Add juice of half a lemon and cook for 1 minute. Sprinkle with feta cheese.

CHEF'S NOTES: Lemon juice adds a vibrant, fresh taste to this dish that has Mediterranean flair and great nutritional value. Adventurous? Try a few sprinkles of red pepper flakes to add a little heat.

Exchanges/Food Choices

1/2 Starch   1 Vegetable   4 Lean Meat

Basic Nutritional Values

Calories	255
Calories from Fat	70
Total Fat	8.0 g
Saturated Fat	2.1 g
Trans Fat	0.0 g
Cholesterol	65 mg
Sodium	305 mg
Potassium	660 mg
Total Carbohydrate	16 g
Dietary Fiber	5 g
Sugars	3 g
Protein	29 g
Phosphorus	300 mg

Thai Chicken Kabobs with Peanut Butter Dipping Sauce

SERVES 4   **SERVING SIZE** 2 kabobs and 1 Tbsp Peanut Butter Dipping Sauce

½ tsp blue agave syrup
       Juice of ½ lime
 1 tsp garlic powder
½ tsp ground black pepper
    4 skinless, boneless chicken breasts
       cut into pieces (24 oz total)
    8 bamboo skewers, soaked in water
       according to directions
4 Tbsp Peanut Butter Dipping Sauce
       (page 121)

1 Combine syrup, lime juice, garlic powder, and pepper.

2 Marinate the chicken pieces in the mixture for 2–3 hours, then thread onto the skewers.

3 Arrange skewers on a baking rack and broil for 4 minutes, turning the kabobs halfway through cooking time.

4 Serve with Peanut Butter Dipping Sauce.

CHEF'S NOTES: Thai cooking, like Jamaican cooking, loves the use of spice and heat. These kabobs are great to serve to guests. Peanuts and peanut butter are often used in this type of cuisine.

Exchanges/Food Choices
5 Lean Meat   1/2 Fat

Basic Nutritional Values

Calories	265
Calories from Fat	90
Total Fat	10.0 g
Saturated Fat	2.1 g
Trans Fat	0.0 g
Cholesterol	95 mg
Sodium	205 mg
Potassium	375 mg
Total Carbohydrate	4 g
Dietary Fiber	1 g
Sugars	2 g
Protein	38 g
Phosphorus	300 mg

Peanut Butter Dipping Sauce

SERVES 24

¾ cup no-sugar-added peanut butter
Juice of 2 limes
2 Tbsp dark sesame oil
1 Tbsp grated ginger
1 tsp onion powder
⅓ cup reduced-sodium soy sauce
1 Tbsp red pepper flakes

1 Combine all ingredients in a saucepan and stir over low heat until the sauce is creamy.

Exchanges/Food Choices
1 1/2 Fat

Basic Nutritional Values

Calories	70
Calories from Fat	45
Total Fat	5.0 g
Saturated Fat	0.9 g
Trans Fat	0.0 g
Cholesterol	0 mg
Sodium	120 mg
Potassium	65 mg
Total Carbohydrate	3 g
Dietary Fiber	1 g
Sugars	1 g
Protein	2 g
Phosphorus	35 mg

Cuban Roasted Pork Loin

SERVES 8

6 Tbsp	olive oil
1	medium onion, grated
5	cloves garlic, mashed
	Juice of 3 limes
¼ cup	orange juice
1 tsp	ground black pepper
2 tsp	oregano
2 tsp	chopped fresh rosemary
2 lb	boneless pork loin, trimmed of visible fat

1. Prepare the marinade by combining all ingredients except the pork in a small saucepan.

2. Stir over low heat until the ingredients combine. Set aside to cool.

3. Pierce the pork loin with a fork and put it in a baking dish.

4. Pour all but 1/4 cup of the marinade over the meat and refrigerate, covered, for 3–5 hours.

5. Roast at 350°F until the meat is no longer pink and juices run clear (it should register 140–145°F on a meat thermometer), about 35 minutes. Baste with the reserved marinade.

CHEF'S NOTES: Roast pork or pernil is a staple of Cuban cooking. Serve leftovers, chopped up in a salad of arugula, tomatoes, and purple onion for a delicious lunch.

Exchanges/Food Choices
1/2 Carbohydrate   3 Lean Meat   2 Fat

Basic Nutritional Values

Calories	260
Calories from Fat	155
Total Fat	17.0 g
Saturated Fat	3.9 g
Trans Fat	0.0 g
Cholesterol	60 mg
Sodium	40 mg
Potassium	325 mg
Total Carbohydrate	4 g
Dietary Fiber	1 g
Sugars	2 g
Protein	21 g
Phosphorus	170 mg

Peppers Stuffed with Rice and Greens

SERVES 6   **SERVING SIZE** 1/2 pepper with filling

3	large green peppers
1 Tbsp	olive oil
	Nonstick cooking spray
6 cups	greens of choice (broccoli greens, kale, collard greens)
1	medium onion, diced
½ cup	chopped green pepper (or another color for contrast)
3	cloves garlic, minced
1 cup	cooked brown rice or cooked quinoa
¼ cup	grated fresh Parmesan cheese
	Salt and pepper, to taste

1. Preheat oven to 400°F.

2. Wash green peppers and cut in half lengthwise, leaving the stem on, to make little "boats." Scrape out pulp and seeds. Brush inside and out with the olive oil.

3. Place peppers, cut-side down, in a 9 × 12-inch baking dish treated with nonstick cooking spray. Bake just until the peppers are soft but not mushy, about 10 minutes. Set aside to cool.

4. While peppers are baking and cooling, prepare the filling. Bring 2 quarts salted water to a boil and add greens. Reduce heat and cover, cooking until the greens are tender (time will vary according to the type of greens you use). Cool slightly and chop into small pieces.

5. Sauté onion, bell pepper, and garlic using a nonstick pan until the onion is golden brown and the mixture is fragrant. Stir in rice and greens.

6. Divide rice/vegetable mixture evenly among the green pepper "boats." Top each "boat" with Parmesan cheese and season with salt and pepper.

7. Pour an inch of water into the bottom of the baking pan and cover with foil. Bake until the peppers and stuffing are warmed up, about 15–20 minutes. Remove the foil and heat an additional 5 minutes uncovered. Serve immediately.

CHEF'S NOTES: Green, red, yellow, orange—peppers come in many colors and many degrees of heat. In this recipe we are using sweet bell peppers. You will find them much more affordable at your farmers market than at the grocery store. These stuffed peppers are full of vitamins C and K.

Exchanges/Food Choices
1/2 Starch   2 Vegetable   1 Fat

Basic Nutritional Values

Calories	125
Calories from Fat	35
Total Fat	4.0 g
Saturated Fat	1.0 g
Trans Fat	0.0 g
Cholesterol	0 mg
Sodium	75 mg
Potassium	465 mg
Total Carbohydrate	20 g
Dietary Fiber	4 g
Sugars	6 g
Protein	5 g
Phosphorus	120 mg

W hat is better than a sweet treat? A sweet treat that is healthy to eat.

There is one ingredient missing from all of the recipes in this chapter—that ingredient is guilt. Don't want it. Don't need it. I'm going to eliminate it from my vocabulary.

Having diabetes does not mean that we have to eliminate dessert from our meal plan. But note one important word: plan. You wouldn't head out on a trip without a plan. As the saying goes, "When we fail to plan, we plan to fail." You and I are not going to fail!

So, as you are deciding what you will have to eat tomorrow, be sure to make room for a light, melt-in-your-mouth Chocolate Almond Meringue Cookie (page 128) or a serving of Fruit Compote with Ginger Cream (page 132).

Walking through the farmers market recently, I saw a young mom pushing a stroller with a little boy who looked to be about four years old. She was trying to keep him from climbing out. The more upset she became, the louder he screamed. "If you sit down and be quiet I'll give you some candy," she said.

Just then the woman who was in charge of one of my favorite farm stands walked over and offered the mom a piece of cheese on a piece of waxed paper and a small red apple. "Would you like these for your little one?" she asked the mom who was red faced by now. The mom smiled and thanked her. Soon the boy was contentedly munching away on his healthy treats.

This is another example of why I treasure farmers markets. There is a sense of small town community there, a degree of caring and concern and connection to one another. That little boy also proved that treats do not have to be full of sugar, carbs, and empty calories to be enjoyable.

That scene was a sweet ending to my visit.

Fresh Figs with Orange Whip

Raspberry Granita

Chocolate Almond Meringue Cookies

Date Baked Apples

Pumpkin "Pies"

Gingered Fruit Salad

Fruit Compote with Ginger Cream

Sparkling Raspberry Lemonade

Non-Dairy Chocolate Pudding

Pumpkin Pudding

Pineapple Cider

Tropical Fruit Mousse

Honey and Cinnamon-Roasted Figs

Maple Walnut Spiced Poached Pears

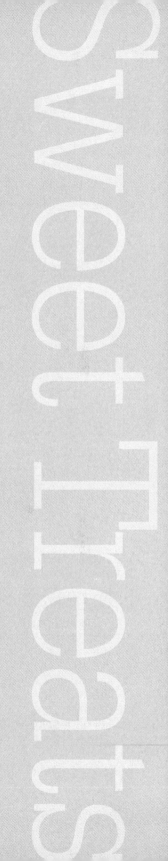

Fresh Figs with Orange Whip

SERVES 8

SERVING SIZE 1/8th recipe

10	fresh figs, peeled and chopped
¼ cup	light whipping cream, whipped
⅓ cup	chopped mandarin orange slices
1 Tbsp	orange extract

1. Place fig pieces in a glass container and pour orange extract over, stirring so all the pieces are coated.

2. Set aside for 1 hour.

3. Combine the whipped cream and mandarin oranges.

4. Fold in the fig pieces.

CHEF'S NOTES: This orange-enhanced, fresh fig whip is full of vitamin C and fiber. If you have tasted figs only in cookies, this dessert will show you just how versatile this fruit can be.

Exchanges/Food Choices
1 Fruit   1/2 Fat

Basic Nutritional Values

Calories	75
Calories from Fat	20
Total Fat	2.5 g
Saturated Fat	1.5 g
Trans Fat	0.0 g
Cholesterol	10 mg
Sodium	0 mg
Potassium	165 mg
Total Carbohydrate	13 g
Dietary Fiber	2 g
Sugars	11 g
Protein	1 g
Phosphorus	15 mg

Raspberry Granita

SERVES 8

SERVING SIZE 1/8th recipe

1½ lb	raspberries (fresh or frozen)
1½ cups	water
2 Tbsp	blue agave syrup
1 tsp	balsamic vinegar

1. Blend the berries to a fine fruit pulp.

2. Add the water, agave syrup, and balsamic vinegar. Add more agave syrup or vinegar to taste.

3. Stir together and pour into a glass or metal 12 × 2-inch baking dish.

4. Cool in freezer until ice crystals form (about 2 hours).

5. Using a fork, stir the chilled mixture to break up the ice crystals and return mixture to the freezer for 30 minutes.

6. Repeat this process and return mixture to the freezer, removing and fork-stirring several times over the course of 4 hours. The finished granita should be light and fluffy.

Exchanges/Food Choices
1 Carbohydrate

Basic Nutritional Values

Calories	60	
Calories from Fat	5	
Total Fat	0.5	g
Saturated Fat	0.0	g
Trans Fat	0.0	g
Cholesterol	0	mg
Sodium	0	mg
Potassium	130	mg
Total Carbohydrate	14	g
Dietary Fiber	6	g
Sugars	7	g
Protein	1	g
Phosphorus	25	mg

CHEF'S NOTES: Easy to prepare. Sweet, tart, and refreshing. Diabetes friendly. What more could we ask for?

Chocolate Almond Meringue Cookies

SERVES 24   **SERVING SIZE** 1 cookie

	Nonstick cooking spray
1 tsp	cornstarch
1 Tbsp	unsweetened cocoa powder
¼ cup	ground almonds (aka "almond meal")
½ cup	granulated sugar, divided use
2	egg whites
¼ tsp	cream of tartar

1. Preheat oven to 250°F.

2. Line 2 cookie sheets with foil and treat with nonstick cooking spray.

3. Mix the cornstarch, cocoa powder, and ground almonds with half the sugar.

4. In a separate bowl, whip the egg whites until foamy and add the cream of tartar. Continue beating until the egg whites form soft peaks. Add the rest of the sugar and continue to beat until the egg white peaks are glossy and stiff.

5. Fold the cocoa/almond mixture into the meringue. Drop by spoonfuls onto the prepared cookie sheets.

6. Bake until the meringues are set and beginning to brown (30–40 minutes). Cool completely. Store in an airtight container.

Exchanges/Food Choices
1/2 Carbohydrate

Basic Nutritional Values

Calories	25
Calories from Fat	5
Total Fat	0.5 g
Saturated Fat	0.1 g
Trans Fat	0.0 g
Cholesterol	0 mg
Sodium	0 mg
Potassium	25 mg
Total Carbohydrate	5 g
Dietary Fiber	0 g
Sugars	4 g
Protein	1 g
Phosphorus	10 mg

CHEF'S NOTES: I admit this is a recipe with quite a few steps, but it is well worth the bit of extra time it might take to prepare. These cookies melt in your mouth, leaving a hint of sweetness and absolutely no guilt. For mocha meringues, add 1 tsp instant coffee.

Date Baked Apples

½ tsp   cinnamon
¼ tsp   nutmeg
¼ tsp   ginger
1 tsp   cornstarch
2 cups   apple juice
¾ cup   chopped dates
1 tsp   vanilla extract
1 tsp   butter
8   medium apples (I use a combination of Golden Delicious and Granny Smith)
2 tsp   lemon juice
½ cup   Splenda Brown Sugar Blend
Nonstick cooking spray

1 Preheat oven to 350°F.

2 In a small saucepan mix together the cinnamon, nutmeg, ginger, and cornstarch. Whisk in apple juice and over medium heat bring to a boil. Stir in dates. Remove from heat, add vanilla and butter.

3 Let the warm mixture sit while you peel, core, and slice apples as you would for pie. Toss apple slices with lemon juice and Splenda Brown Sugar Blend.

4 Place the apples into a greased baking pan (use nonstick cooking spray) and pour the date and juice mixture over the top.

5 Bake for 30 minutes or until apples are tender.

CHEF'S NOTES: Don't buy dates mixed with sugar. Buy whole dates and chop them yourself. You can use kitchen shears to make cutting up the dates even easier. I like to make this sweet and spicy dessert any time of the year. During the holiday season I splurge a little and use fresh dates and sprinkle 1/4 cup of chopped nuts on top before serving.

Exchanges/Food Choices
1 1/2 Fruit   1/2 Carbohydrate

Basic Nutritional Values

Calories	120
Calories from Fat	5
Total Fat	0.5 g
Saturated Fat	0.2 g
Trans Fat	0.0 g
Cholesterol	0 mg
Sodium	5 mg
Potassium	190 mg
Total Carbohydrate	31 g
Dietary Fiber	2 g
Sugars	22 g
Protein	1 g
Phosphorus	20 mg

Pumpkin "Pies"

SERVES 8

1	(15- to 16-oz) can pumpkin
2	eggs, slightly beaten
½ **tsp**	ground cloves
½ **tsp**	ground ginger
½ **tsp**	nutmeg
½ **tsp**	cinnamon
2 **tsp**	brown sugar substitute
1	(12-oz) can skim or low-fat evaporated milk
6	sugar-free oatmeal cookies (for example, Murray Sugar Free Oatmeal cookies)

1 Combine all ingredients except the oatmeal cookies, mix, and pour into 8 glass ramekins.

2 Bake at 325°F for 25 minutes or until set.

3 Check to see if "pies" are done by inserting a knife. When it comes out clean they are done.

4 Crumble cookies and sprinkle over the pumpkin.

CHEF'S NOTES: Substituting the oatmeal cookies for the usual pie crust adds fiber and cuts calories and fat. Sometimes I add 1 tsp of nonfat vanilla yogurt on top. There are some excellent high-fiber, diabetes-friendly cookies for sale. Choose a small box and freeze the cookies you do not use for this recipe so you won't be tempted to eat more than you know you should!

Exchanges/Food Choices
1 Carbohydrate   1/2 Fat

Basic Nutritional Values

Calories	115
Calories from Fat	30
Total Fat	3.5 g
Saturated Fat	1.2 g
Trans Fat	0.0 g
Cholesterol	50 mg
Sodium	110 mg
Potassium	300 mg
Total Carbohydrate	16 g
Dietary Fiber	2 g
Sugars	8 g
Protein	6 g
Phosphorus	140 mg

Gingered Fruit Salad

SALAD

2	medium just-ripe bananas, cut into thick chunks
2 Tbsp	lemon juice
2	medium navel oranges, peeled and cut into thin rounds
1	medium papaya, peeled, seeded, and chopped into chunks
1	medium pineapple, cut into chunks (may use canned in juice)

GINGER DRESSING

1 cup	plain, low-fat yogurt
1 Tbsp	honey
1 Tbsp	chopped candied ginger

1. Toss the banana pieces in the lemon juice so they don't turn brown.

2. Mix the fruit in a large bowl and divide onto individual plates.

3. Stir all dressing ingredients together. Serve salad with ginger dressing.

CHEF'S NOTES: Banana, papaya, and pineapple with a bit of ginger to enhance their flavors—you will think you are in the Islands!

Exchanges/Food Choices
1 Fruit   1/2 Carbohydrate

Basic Nutritional Values

Calories	95
Calories from Fat	5
Total Fat	0.5 g
Saturated Fat	0.3 g
Trans Fat	0.0 g
Cholesterol	0 mg
Sodium	20 mg
Potassium	325 mg
Total Carbohydrate	23 g
Dietary Fiber	2 g
Sugars	16 g
Protein	2 g
Phosphorus	55 mg

Fruit Compote with Ginger Cream

SERVES 6   **SERVING SIZE** 1/2 cup compote

COMPOTE

3 cups	fresh peaches, washed and coarsely chopped with the skin on
½ cup	water (more if necessary)
1 Tbsp	blue agave syrup
1 Tbsp	fresh lemon juice
1 tsp	ground ginger
½ tsp	cinnamon
¼ tsp	ground cloves (optional)

GINGER CREAM

1 cup	plain, nonfat yogurt
2 Tbsp	nonfat milk
1 Tbsp	blue agave syrup
1	piece crystallized ginger, very finely chopped (about 1 tsp)

1 Combine all compote ingredients in a medium saucepan and cook over low heat, stirring occasionally, until the fruit is soft. Add more water if the mixture is too thick.

2 Whisk all ginger cream ingredients together. If sauce is too thick, thin it with a little more milk. Refrigerate until ready to serve.

3 Spoon compote into individual serving bowls while warm and top each serving with a spoonful of the ginger cream.

4 Serve immediately.

CHEF'S NOTES: I love to use completely ripe, juicy freestone peaches in this recipe. You can substitute a combination of stone fruits—peaches, nectarines, plums, or apricots—for this recipe, but don't use cherries. I know I say ground cloves are optional but I would never leave them out. And the ginger cream is so delicious you will want to eat it all by itself.

Exchanges/Food Choices
1 Carbohydrate

Basic Nutritional Values

Calories	80
Calories from Fat	0
Total Fat	0.0 g
Saturated Fat	0.1 g
Trans Fat	0.0 g
Cholesterol	0 mg
Sodium	30 mg
Potassium	260 mg
Total Carbohydrate	17 g
Dietary Fiber	1 g
Sugars	15 g
Protein	3 g
Phosphorus	85 mg

Sparkling Raspberry Lemonade

SERVES 10

SERVING SIZE 1/2 cup

6	large lemons
½ cup	Splenda granulated
1 cup	unsweetened raspberries (fresh or frozen)
1 quart	very cold sparkling water

1 Mix the juice of 6 lemons with the Splenda.

2 Add the raspberries and mix lightly so that the berries don't break.

3 Chill the mixture in the freezer until it's slushy.

4 Spoon mixture into a pitcher and then pour in the cold sparkling water.

CHEF'S NOTES: Raspberries are delicate little nuggets full of flavor and vitamin C. When they are available at my farmers market, I freeze them on a cookie sheet, bag them, and put them right back into the freezer. This lemonade is a dessert in a glass that I like to sip slowly while sitting outside enjoying the beauty of nature.

Exchanges/Food Choices
Free food

Basic Nutritional Values

Calories	15	
Calories from Fat	0	
Total Fat	0.0	g
Saturated Fat	0.0	g
Trans Fat	0.0	g
Cholesterol	0	mg
Sodium	10	mg
Potassium	45	mg
Total Carbohydrate	4	g
Dietary Fiber	1	g
Sugars	2	g
Protein	0	g
Phosphorus	5	mg

Non-Dairy Chocolate Pudding

SERVES 4

SERVING SIZE 1/4 recipe

1	(1-lb) package soft silken tofu, drained
2 Tbsp	cocoa powder
1 Tbsp	blue agave syrup
¼ cup	Splenda granulated
½ tsp	almond extract (or 1 tsp vanilla extract)
⅛ tsp	salt

1 Combine all ingredients in a blender.

2 Chill for 3 hours before serving.

CHEF'S NOTES: Silken tofu brings a boost of protein and a smooth texture to this pudding. Tofu takes on the flavors it is mixed with, so you will taste nothing but cocoa/almond sweetness.

Exchanges/Food Choices
1/2 Carbohydrate   1 Lean Meat

Basic Nutritional Values

Calories	90
Calories from Fat	30
Total Fat	3.5 g
Saturated Fat	0.6 g
Trans Fat	0.0 g
Cholesterol	0 mg
Sodium	80 mg
Potassium	245 mg
Total Carbohydrate	10 g
Dietary Fiber	1 g
Sugars	7 g
Protein	6 g
Phosphorus	90 mg

Pumpkin Pudding

1 cup	pumpkin purée
1	package instant, sugar-free vanilla pudding mix
1 tsp	pumpkin pie spice
1 cup	evaporated skim milk
1 cup	nonfat milk

1 Blend ingredients until smooth.

2 Chill for several hours before serving.

CHEF'S NOTES: You can make your own pumpkin pie spice by mixing cinnamon, nutmeg, cloves, and ginger. Talk to farmers market stand holders to find the best pumpkin for cooking and puréeing. I have substituted butternut squash for the pumpkin in the past. Whichever you use, just cut it in half, bake, and scrape out the soft interior. Add a sprinkle of nutmeg on the top of this pudding.

Exchanges/Food Choices
1/2 Fat-Free Milk   1/2 Carbohydrate

Basic Nutritional Values

Calories	80
Calories from Fat	0
Total Fat	0.0 g
Saturated Fat	0.2 g
Trans Fat	0.0 g
Cholesterol	5 mg
Sodium	270 mg
Potassium	295 mg
Total Carbohydrate	14 g
Dietary Fiber	1 g
Sugars	8 g
Protein	5 g
Phosphorus	255 mg

Pineapple Cider

SERVES 10

SERVING SIZE 1/10th recipe

2 cups   unsweetened pineapple juice
4 cups   unsweetened apple cider
1 tsp   powdered ginger
½ cup   fresh mint leaves
1   (28-oz) bottle diet ginger ale
         (room temperature)

1. Combine the juice and the cider in a medium saucepan. Add the powdered ginger.

2. Crush the mint and add to the juices.

3. Bring to a boil.

4. Strain out the mint. Add the ginger ale.

5. Serve immediately.

CHEF'S NOTES: You can refrigerate the mixture (before adding ginger ale) and use only enough for 1 serving at a time. Keep the ginger ale chilled and add to each glass as needed. This drink is very high in vitamin C. Some days I enjoy this with breakfast.

Exchanges/Food Choices
1 Fruit

Basic Nutritional Values

Calories	75
Calories from Fat	0
Total Fat	0.0 g
Saturated Fat	0.0 g
Trans Fat	0.0 g
Cholesterol	0 mg
Sodium	10 mg
Potassium	185 mg
Total Carbohydrate	18 g
Dietary Fiber	1 g
Sugars	15 g
Protein	0 g
Phosphorus	15 mg

Tropical Fruit Mousse

2	medium mangos, peeled, seeded, and cubed
1	medium guava (about 3 ¾ oz), peeled, seeded, and cubed
1	medium banana, cut into chunks
¾ cup	plain, nonfat yogurt
2 tsp	honey
6	ice cubes
1 tsp	vanilla extract

1. Combine all ingredients in a blender and blend until smooth.

2. Refrigerate for at least 3 hours before spooning into serving dishes.

CHEF'S NOTES: If you are unable to find guava just add an extra mango.

Exchanges/Food Choices
1 Fruit   1/2 Carbohydrate

Basic Nutritional Values

Calories	105
Calories from Fat	0
Total Fat	0.0 g
Saturated Fat	0.1 g
Trans Fat	0.0 g
Cholesterol	0 mg
Sodium	20 mg
Potassium	325 mg
Total Carbohydrate	24 g
Dietary Fiber	3 g
Sugars	19 g
Protein	2 g
Phosphorus	65 mg

Honey and Cinnamon-Roasted Figs

SERVES 5

SERVING SIZE 2 figs and about 2 Tbsp yogurt

10	figs
2 Tbsp	clear honey
2–4 tsp	cinnamon
½ cup	plain, non-fat Greek-style yogurt

1. Preheat oven to 400°F or heat broiler.

2. Cut a cross in the top of each fig, pierce through the stem but not through the base, so that the pieces remain intact. Place into a shallow ovenproof dish, pulling them open gently as you do. Drizzle the honey over the insides of the figs and sprinkle with cinnamon.

3. Bake or broil for about 15 minutes or until the figs are tender but not collapsed. Serve with Greek-style yogurt.

CHEF'S NOTES: Too often the flavor and nutritional value of the fig is underestimated. The succulent sweetness of fig combined with its high fiber content, potassium, and iron levels make this powerhouse a must-have in a healthy diet.

Exchanges/Food Choices
1 1/2 Fruit   1/2 Carbohydrate

Basic Nutritional Values

Calories	115	
Calories from Fat	0	
Total Fat	0.0	g
Saturated Fat	0.1	g
Trans Fat	0.0	g
Cholesterol	0	mg
Sodium	10	mg
Potassium	265	mg
Total Carbohydrate	28	g
Dietary Fiber	3	g
Sugars	24	g
Protein	3	g
Phosphorus	45	mg

Maple Walnut Spiced Poached Pears

SERVES 4   **SERVING SIZE** 2 pear halves, 1 Tbsp chopped nuts, and 1 Tbsp poaching liquid

4	medium ripe pears
2 cups	water
	Juice of 1 lemon
3	whole cloves
1	stick cinnamon
2 Tbsp	maple syrup
4 Tbsp	finely chopped walnuts

1 Cut pears in half. Remove core.

2 Put water, lemon juice, cloves, cinnamon, and maple syrup in a large pan. Add pears cut-side down. Cover and simmer until pears are softened but not mushy.

3 Put pears into shallow dish with half of the poaching liquid.

4 To serve place 2 halves onto plate. Drizzle 1 Tbsp of poaching liquid on top of the pears. Sprinkle with chopped walnuts.

CHEF'S NOTES: I suggest using pure maple syrup in this recipe. It is a bit more expensive but a small amount will give a more intense flavor.

Exchanges/Food Choices
2 Fruit   1 Fat

Basic Nutritional Values

Calories	160
Calories from Fat	45
Total Fat	5.0 g
Saturated Fat	0.5 g
Trans Fat	0.0 g
Cholesterol	0 mg
Sodium	0 mg
Potassium	245 mg
Total Carbohydrate	30 g
Dietary Fiber	6 g
Sugars	20 g
Protein	2 g
Phosphorus	45 mg

Beyond the Farmers Market

By shopping at a farmers market you help support the hard-working owners of small farms who are committed to providing you with healthy products for a healthy lifestyle. If you are interested in becoming even more involved in the process, check into Community Supported Agriculture (CSA). Visit http://www.nal.usda.gov/afsic/pubs/csa/csa.shtml to learn more about the process and find opportunities in your area. When you are a member of a CSA, you purchase a share of the produce from a local farm. Each week during the growing season you will receive your share of the fruits, herbs, and vegetables being harvested. This is a great opportunity to try some foods you haven't eaten before. Your farmer will be happy to give you ideas on how to use these new-to-you ingredients. In some cases you and your family might have the opportunity to reduce the amount you pay by helping out on the farm. This is a chance to enjoy family fun and move your bodies!

Another treasure is your local Extension Office. The Cooperative Extension System is ready to help you make the most of your farmers market purchases. Through this system you can learn about everything from the growing season in your area to how to choose the best produce and much more. The Cooperative Extension System has offices throughout the nation. Experts offer written information, educational opportunities, and answers to questions about living a healthier life. Visit http://www.nifa.usda.gov/Extension/index.html to access a searchable map that will guide you to the Cooperative Extension

System office closest to you. Most of their services are free but there may be a few classes with a small fee.

Your Cooperative Extension office can also help you connect the young people in your life with the 4-H program. Many people mistakenly believe that 4-H is only for rural areas. Not true! There are chapters across the country from big cities to the suburbs to farming communities. And 4-H is not just about agriculture and raising animals, it is about learning to be healthy in all areas of your life.

Their pledge—

> I pledge my head to clearer thinking,
> My heart to greater loyalty,
> My hands to larger service,
> and my health to better living,
> for my club, my community, my country, and my world.

—is very important for people with (and without) diabetes. The new lifestyle our bodies demand calls for clearer thinking and loyalty to the rules we must follow to live better, healthier lives. As we commit ourselves to sharing what we learn, we inspire those around us to learn about diabetes. This is how we will fight this disease.

List of Recipes

Subject Index

Cuban Black Bean Soup, 36
Curried Leek and Lentil Soup, 24
Grand Green Gazpacho, 26
Jade Soup, 28
Luscious Low-Carb Tortilla Soup, 31
Mmmm Mushroom Soup, 27
Summer Sour Cherry Soup, 23
Tomato Mushroom Soup, 34
2, 2, 2 Good Gazpacho, 30
soy nut, 76
Sparkling Raspberry Lemonade, 133
sparkling water, 133
Spiced Sweet Potato Fries, 86
Spicy Asian Vinaigrette, 50
Spicy Asian Vinaigrette, 56
Spicy Fish and Collard Greens, 98
Spicy Lentil and Sausage Stew, 35
Spicy Skinny Slaw, 50
spinach, 28, 40, 49, 53, 64, 74, 79, 107–108
Spinach-Wrapped Chicken, 108
split pea, 81
squash, 33, 48, 82
stew
    Chicken Barley Stew, 22
    Easy Seafood Stew, 25
    Moroccan Lamb Stew with Apricots, 116
    Spicy Lentil and Sausage Stew, 35
Stir-Fried Snow Peas, 80
Stir-Fried Spicy Greens, 74
Stone Soup, 20
strawberries, 7–8, 40
sugar, 17
Summer of Ben Tyler (Hallmark), 37
Summer Sour Cherry Soup, 23
sunflower seed, 6, 48–49, 73, 76
Sunflower Soy "Butter", 76
Sweet and Smoky Baked Eggs, 10
sweet potato, 86, 89, 92

sweet treat
    Chocolate Almond Meringue Cookies, 128
    Date Baked Apples, 129
    Fresh Figs with Orange Whip, 126
    Fruit Compote with Ginger Cream, 132
    Gingered Fruit Salad, 131
    Honey and Cinnamon-Roasted Figs, 138
    Maple Walnut Spiced Poached Pears, 139
    Non-Dairy Chocolate Pudding, 134
    Pineapple Cider, 136
    Pumpkin "Pies", 130
    Pumpkin Pudding, 135
    Raspberry Granita, 127
    Sparkling Raspberry Lemonade, 133
    Tropical Fruit Mousse, 137

T
Tabbouleh Salad, 39
Tangy Green Beans, 84
Thai Chicken Kabobs with Peanut Butter Dipping
    Sauce, 120
thyme, 87
tips, 16
tofu, 28, 134
tomato, 30, 78–79, 81, 99
    beefsteak, 10, 68, 82, 89
    cherry, 114
    Chickpea, Tomato, and Cilantro Salad with
        Peanuts, 41
    paste, 22, 66, 113
    Roma, 31, 46, 55, 104
    stewed, 34
    Tomato Mushroom Soup, 34
    Tomato-Cucumber Salad with Lemon Juice, 44
    yellow, 26
tortilla, 31, 114
Tropical Fruit Mousse, 137
turkey, 96, 115